CW00377033

Dental Materials in Operative Dentistry

Quintessentials of Dental Practice – 33
Operative Dentistry – 5

Dental Materials in Operative Dentistry

By

Christina A Mitchell

Editor-in-Chief: Nairn H F Wilson
Editor Operative Dentistry: Paul A Brunton

Quintessence Publishing Co. Ltd.
London, Berlin, Chicago, Paris, Milan, Barcelona, Istanbul,
São Paulo, Tokyo, New Delhi, Moscow, Prague, Warsaw

British Library Cataloguing in Publication Data

Mitchell, Christina A.
   Dental materials in operative dentistry. - (Quintessentials of dental practice; v. 33)
   1. Dental materials
   I. Title
   617.6'95

ISBN-13: 9781850971290

ISBN-13: 978-1-85097-129-0

Foreword

Good knowledge and understanding of dental materials is fundamental to favourable clinical outcomes in the practice of dentistry. Given that the restoration of teeth continues to comprise 60–70% of dental care, the importance to success in practice of a sound knowledge and understanding of the nature, selection and effective application of restorative materials is self-evident.

This addition to the unique *Quintessentials of Dental Practice* series is yet another jewel in the crown. It is no easy matter to make applied dental materials science engaging and enjoyable, in particular to a wide audience ranging from student to experienced practitioner. This volume has achieved this goal in exemplary fashion, with the added benefit of lots of authoritative advice and guidance of immediate practical relevance. If you are not up to speed with the large array of new and alternative forms of direct restorative materials and related products and procedures, this book is a "must", not to be put down and left gnawing at your conscience.

Yes, this book has all the hallmarks of a carefully planned and crafted *Quintessentials* volume – easy and quick to read, nicely illustrated and a great source of essential information. Considerable skill, let alone meticulous attention, has gone into planning, preparing and producing this book to give it the necessary appeal to its intended audience.

The restoration of teeth is an art and a science. Without the necessary knowledge and understanding, there is no scientific appreciation and, in turn, the art is flawed. This excellent book is an effective key to essential scientific understanding and, as a consequence, a portal to new opportunities and professional fulfilment in the art of modern operative dentistry.

Nairn Wilson
Editor-in-Chief

Preface

The subject of dental materials has long been considered a dull, but necessary area of study by dental undergraduate students. However, upon graduation, dentists discover that the field is fast-changing, and that the ability to discriminate between "hype" and reality is both professionally and financially essential.

The world of dental materials is inhabited by clinicians, engineers, material scientists, polymer scientists, chemists, metallurgists and cellular biologists, all of whose skills are required to conceive, develop and test new materials and devices. Recent advances in adhesive dentistry now permit clinical procedures that were impossible only a few years ago. Significant problem areas remain, such as microleakage of adhesive bonds and the biocompatibility of all dental materials, so there is still plenty of opportunity for future research.

The aim of this book is to summarise, in a concise fashion, current knowledge of dental materials used in operative dentistry. I have tried to achieve a balance between clinical relevance and the underlying scientific data.

The names of commercially available dental materials are given in this book. Of necessity, the materials cited are not comprehensive and, inevitably, will date rapidly as manufacturers develop and market new materials. To help counteract this intrinsic obsolescence, I have included a list of dental manufacturer websites, which provide up-to-date information on dental products. In addition, for those readers wishing to delve deeper into particular topics, selected references are provided at the end of each chapter.

Christina A Mitchell

Acknowledgements

Publishing a book is a team effort and requires the skills of many people, whom I wish to thank.

To Robert Thompson, for his expertise and attention to detail in producing the excellent quality photographs. I am greatly indebted to him for his commitment to this project. His work has immeasurably enhanced the presentation of this book.

To Brian, Sarah and Rachel, for their support, patience and understanding during the many days spent in the preparation of this book.

And finally, thank you to my friends, colleagues and mentors in the worlds of dental materials research and clinical dentistry for their inspiration and motivation.

Contents

Chapter 1
Resin Composites

Aim

The aim of this chapter is to improve understanding of the wide range of resin composites (including ormocers and ceromers) available for the restoration of anterior and posterior teeth.

Outcome

Readers will gain knowledge of the advantages and disadvantages of each of the many different types of resin composite materials available and how properties relate to material composition.

Introduction

Resin composites may be used to restore anterior and posterior teeth. When used anteriorly, aesthetics are often of primary concern, requiring durable high surface polish, excellent colour matching and colour stability. Posteriorly, where biting forces may be up to 600 N, high compressive and tensile strength and excellent wear resistance are required. Both anterior and posterior resin composites require a reliable bond to enamel and dentine to prevent leakage between the tooth and the restoration and to provide dimensional stability. Resin composites were first used in dentistry in the 1960s, and since then many different types of material have been developed for varying clinical indications.

Indications

Anterior Composites
Resin composite is used as a direct restorative material for the replacement of missing dentine and enamel. It is also used to alter the shape and colour of anterior teeth to enhance aesthetics. It can be used to close diastemas and alter crown length and contour, and it can be placed as a labial veneer to mask intrinsic discolouration and structural defects in a tooth.

Posterior Composites

Resin composite is also increasingly used as a direct restorative material for the replacement of missing dentine and enamel in posterior teeth. It is chosen as an aesthetic alternative to dental amalgam as a definitive restorative material for load-bearing occlusal and proximal preparations, for the restoration of tooth wear and as a core build-up material. It can also be used indirectly, to produce laboratory-made inlays and onlays that are then bonded to the prepared tooth using a resin composite luting cement and dentine adhesive systems. Increasing numbers of patients are requesting alternatives to dental amalgam in response to much-publicised concerns regarding the effects of mercury released from dental amalgam (see Chapter 5, pages 80-81, Safe use and disposal). Resin composite is not, however, an ideal restorative material in all clinical situations.

Composition of Resin Composites

Resin composite comprises resin matrix and glass filler particles, which polymerise (set) by chemical or light initiation. The glass filler particles are coated with a coupling agent to improve the bond to the matrix. In addition, initiators and accelerators are required for polymerisation. Inorganic oxide pigments are added in small amounts to achieve the various shades required.

Resin Matrix

Most resin composites are based on bisphenol-A-glycidyl methacrylate (bis-GMA) or urethane dimethacrylate (UDMA). Other resins used to alter viscosity and handling include triethylene glycol dimethacrylate (TEGDMA) and bisphenol-A-polyethylene glycol diether dimethacrylate.

Glass Filler Particles

Various filler particles are used by dental manufacturers, including silicon dioxide, aluminium oxide, barium, zirconium oxide, borosilicate and barium aluminium silicate glasses. The greater the amount of filler particles, the better the physical and mechanical properties of the material, up to a maximum level. Beyond this, the resin becomes too viscous to use clinically.

Filler particles give the following properties:
• increased wear resistance
• increased hardness
• increased translucency
• decreased polymerisation contraction
• decreased coefficient of thermal expansion.

Resin composites may be classified according to the size and distribution of the filler particles (Table 1-1).

Coupling Agents

Silanes are the most commonly used coupling agents, for example 3-methacryloxypropyl trimethoxysilane (MPS). In many resin composites, the molecule has silanol groups at one end and methacrylate groups at the other. These molecules form covalent bonds to the silicon–oxygen groups of the filler particles and the methacrylate groups of the resin (Ferracane, 1995). When silane is deposited on the filler particle, the methoxy groups hydrolyse to hydroxy groups, which react with water or hydroxyl-radical groups on the filler. The carbon double bonds of the silane react with the resin and form a continuous bond between the filler particles and the resin matrix via the coupling agent. These bonds degrade when exposed to water intraorally (Powers and Sakaguchi, 2006).

Initiators and Accelerators

The majority of resin composites are light-cured. Polymerisation is initiated when the material is exposed to a blue light with a wavelength of around 470 nm. The light is absorbed by a photoactivator, often camphorquinone, which together with an aromatic amine initiates the polymerisation reaction.

Some resin composites are dual-cured, where polymerisation is commenced by exposure to blue light but the reaction continues after light exposure by

Table 1-1 **Classification of resin composites**

Classification	Range of particle sizes (μm)	Filler (% by volume)
Hybrid	0.04–3.0	60–70
Microfill	0.04–0.2	32–50
Condensable (packable)	0.04, 0.2–20	59–80
Flowable	0.04, 0.2–3.0	42–62
Nanohybrid (nanocomposite)	0.002–0.075	68–78.5

the chemical reaction taking place between an organic amine and organic peroxide. This reaction produces free radicals, which react with the carbon double bonds of the resin, causing polymerisation and set of the material. Dual-cured resin composites are useful materials as core materials, where bulk placement may mean that light cannot penetrate to the full depth of the material, and thus the chemical reaction, which proceeds in the absence of light, ensures maximum polymerisation. They are also useful as luting agents for the cementation of all-ceramic crowns, porcelain-fused-to-metal crowns, posts and orthodontic brackets, all situations where full light penetration is not, or may not be, possible.

The amount of polymerisation, or degree of conversion of carbon double bonds to single bonds, varies: typically 65–80% when light-cured and 60–75% when chemically cured. Dual-cured materials may achieve up to 80% degree of conversion. The degree of conversion is clinically relevant because many of the physical and mechanical properties improve as it increases. The degree of polymerisation is affected by the length of time of exposure to the curing light, distance from the curing light, shade of composite, type of resin and filler composition.

The polymerisation reaction produces a net shrinkage of the material as the cross-linkage proceeds. The larger the volume of filler particles in a resin composite, the lower will be the shrinkage, thus microfilled composites, which have the lowest percentage volume of filler particles (Table 1-1), give the highest values of linear shrinkage: 2–3%. Hybrid composites have lower values of linear shrinkage: 0.6–1.4%.

Types of Resin Composite

Microfill Composites

Microfill resin composites are designed for use in anterior preparations, where aesthetics are the primary concern. Traditionally, they have very small silica filler particles, but the particles tend to agglomerate giving very low filler loading, and therefore low strength and wear resistance, and high polymerisation contraction, thermal expansion and water absorption. The small particle size provides good surface polish compared with resin composites with larger filler particles.

Hybrid Composites

Hybrid composites were developed as "universal" materials, with sufficiently good aesthetics to be used anteriorly but with sufficient strength and wear resistance to be also used posteriorly. Some hybrid composites are marketed specifically for posterior use. A typical hybrid composite material is shown in Fig 1-1.

The clinical placement of a hybrid composite material in a distal cavity in an upper right central incisor tooth is illustrated in Figs 1-2 to 1-11.

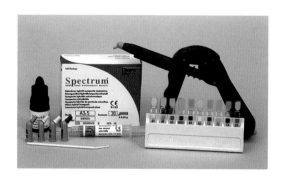

Fig 1-1 Presentation of a typical hybrid resin composite restorative material, showing the enamel and dentine adhesive system, single-use compules, etchant, shade guide and applicator gun.

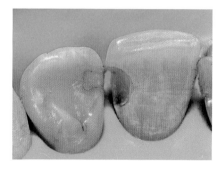

Fig 1-2 Prepared cavity on distal aspect of upper right central incisor tooth. The tooth has been isolated with a rubber dam to prevent contamination of the dentine and enamel by saliva, gingival exudate or blood.

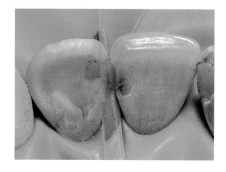

Fig 1-3 Prepared cavity with interproximal acetate matrix strip and wooden wedge in place. The wedge separates the teeth slightly to ensure a tight contact point between the new restoration and the adjacent tooth when the matrix strip is removed. The enamel and dentine of the cavity is then etched with orthophosphoric acid, rinsed and lightly dried.

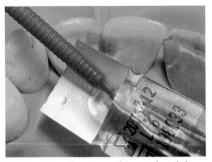

Fig 1-4 Application of enamel and dentine adhesive to a small applicator brush from the product delivery system.

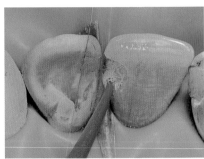

Fig 1-5 Enamel and dentine adhesive system is applied to the etched enamel and dentine with the small applicator brush.

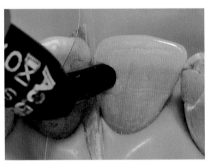

Fig 1-6 Syringing hybrid composite into cavity.

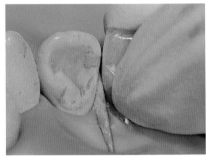

Fig 1-7 Tightly adapting matrix strip around tooth using finger pressure.

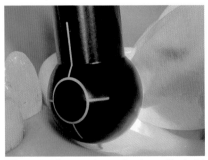

Fig 1-8 Photopolymerisation of hybrid composite material.

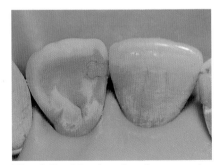

Fig 1-9 Newly placed composite restoration.

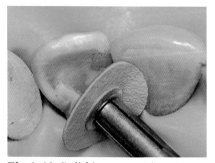

Fig 1-10 Polishing composite restoration with small-diameter aluminium oxide disc.

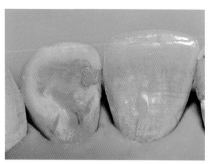

Fig 1-11 Finished hybrid composite material restoration.

Hybrid materials contain a range of particle sizes (Table 1-1), which permits higher filler loading and improved physical properties. The larger filler particles give a poorer surface polish than microfills, so they are not indicated where aesthetics are paramount. In recent years the trend has been to introduce increasingly smaller filler particles, in the spaces between the larger filler particles, to improve the surface polish and maintain filler loading. These materials are referred to as microhybrid resin composites. The most recent resin composites have continued the trend towards smaller filler particles with the use of fillers in the nanometre (10^{-9}) range. These are referred to as nanohybrids or nanocomposites.

Nanocomposites
In general, nanocomposites are recommended for use in direct anterior and posterior restorations, core build-ups, veneers, splinting, inlays and onlays. A number of manufacturers produce nanocomposites; an example of a nanocomposite is shown in Fig 1-12. The main advantages claimed for incorporation of nanofillers are:

- Higher filler loading, giving enhanced physical properties, without increasing viscosity to an unacceptable level.
- High polish can be achieved and maintained long term, giving good aesthetics for anterior use.
- Increased wear resistance.
- Reduced volumetric shrinkage (1.5–1.7%) compared with other resin composite, aiming to reduce residual stress following photo-polymerisation.

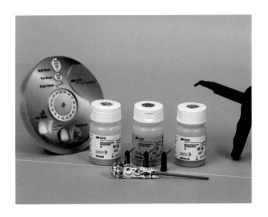

Fig 1-12 A nanocomposite resin composite material, showing the shade guide, compules, enamel and dentine adhesive system and applicator gun.

There is still only a relatively limited amount of independent research on these materials, and further investigation and longer-term clinical trials are required to determine if the above claims are justified.

Several manufacturers combine two to three different types and sizes of fillers in nanocomposites, at least one of which will be in the nanometre range. The resin components of these materials are similar to those of their hybrid resin composite predecessors. One material (Premise, Kerr) contains prepolymerised filler (30–50 μm), barium glass (0.4 μm) and silica nanoparticles (20 nm) with filler (84% by weight or 71.2% by volume).

Another material (Filtek Supreme, 3M ESPE) contains two novel nanoparticles, described as silica "nanomers" (20 nm) and loosely bound agglomerates called "nanoclusters" of zirconia and silica particles (0.6–1.4 μm), giving filler loading of 78.5% (weight). A third material (EsthetX, Dentsply) contains titanium dioxide, silica (40 nm) and barium boron fluoro–aluminosilicate glass (1 μm) filler particles.

Flowable Composites

Flowable composites are reduced-viscosity materials that flow easily and are good at wetting the surface of the preparation (Fig 1-13). These materials have reduced filler loading to reduce viscosity and therefore demonstrate higher polymerisation contraction and wear values and reduced physical properties. They are therefore not suitable for load-bearing restorations. Some materials have compositions similar to the hybrid resin composite produced by the same manufacturer and, most recently, new versions similar

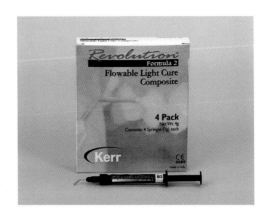

Fig 1-13 A flowable resin composite material, showing the fine applicator tip, which aids placement of this low-viscosity material in narrow cavities.

to the nanocomposite. This low viscosity is achieved by having a low volume of filler particles (Table 1-1).

These composites are useful materials for certain repair and refurbishment procedures. Repairs often involve a narrow slit-shaped preparation or space, which is difficult to restore with a more viscous hybrid or microfill resin composite. The use of a flowable composite to repair a defective cervical resin composite restoration is illustrated in Figs 1-14 to 1-18. Flowable

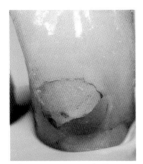

Fig 1-14 A defective resin composite cervical restoration on the labial aspect of a lower left canine tooth.

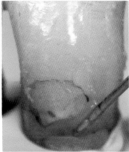

Fig 1-15 Orthophosphoric acid etchant being applied to the dentine and enamel of the area to be repaired. The etchant is then washed and lightly dried.

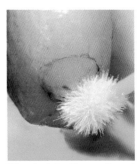

Fig 1-16 Enamel and dentine adhesive system being applied to the cavity with an applicator brush.

9

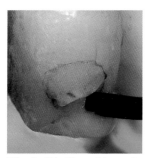 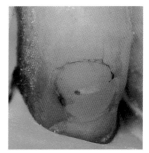

Fig 1-17 Flowable resin composite material being syringed into the area to be repaired. The material is then photopolymerised, shaped and polished.

Fig 1-18 Finished flowable resin composite repair.

composites may also be used as a lining material to block out undercuts when a preparation is to be restored by an indirect method. The majority of flowable composites are not useful as definitive filling materials as they have a tendency to slump prior to polymerisation. It has been suggested, however, that they are useful materials for the restoration of non-carious cervical lesions, as their relatively low modulus of elasticity (lower rigidity) may mean that as the tooth flexes in parafunctional activities (bruxism) the restoration will be able to flex also. A more rigid material will concentrate stress at the tooth–restoration interface, predisposing the restoration to debond. In addition, flowable composites cannot be used in high load-bearing areas (occlusal, proximal and incisal edge preparations) as their low volume of filler particles confers reduced strength and wear resistance compared with other types of resin composites. The majority of flowable composites are light-cured only, which limits their use to areas where light can penetrate.

Flowable resin composites have been suggested as a lining material, under posterior resin composite restorations, to act as a flexible stress-breaker, allowing some relaxation of the stress generated by polymerisation contraction of the posterior resin composite. Flowable composites are less rigid than hybrid or packable composites, used to restore posterior preparations, given their lower filler content, and thus can deform plastically, reducing the likelihood that polymerisation shrinkage stress will break the adhesive bond to the tooth substance. However, the lower filler content causes the flowable composite to undergo greater polymerisation contraction than the more highly filled hybrid or packable composites, which may counteract any hypothetical advantages. Research quantifying leakage under posterior composite restorations has given equivocal results, with some results indicating a reduction in microleakage when flowable composites are used, and others showing no change or an increase in leakage. Reported differences may be related to differences between materials, lining thickness and whether the lining was precured or co-cured with the restorative resin composite. All of these factors will alter the stress distribution at the restoration–tooth interface. Research has, however, clearly indicated that the use of a resin-modified glass-ionomer cement as a liner under posterior composites reduces leakage.

Packable Composites

Packable or condensable composites are high-viscosity materials designed for the restoration of posterior preparations subjected to significant occlusal loading (Fig 1-19). Typically, packable composites have the highest percentage filler volume, conferring low wear rates, reduced polymerisation shrinkage (0.6–0.9%) and increased rigidity. In addition, radiopacifiers are added to aid the radiographical diagnosis of secondary caries, which may be difficult to diagnose clinically in posterior teeth.

Initially, packable composites materials were designed to mimic the ability of dental amalgam to be placed or condensed into a preparation, in an attempt to achieve good adaptation of the composite material to all areas of the preparation, including undercuts, and to facilitate tight proximal contacts. Most clinicians now accept that the handling and placement of a resin composite has little, if anything, in common with the placement of an amalgam and requires the acquisition of different skills. The clinical placement of a packable resin composite restoration is illustrated in Figs 1-20 to 1-29.

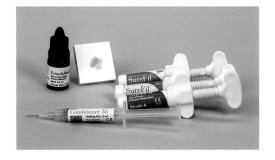

Fig 1-19 Example of a packable resin composite material, designed for restoration of posterior teeth.

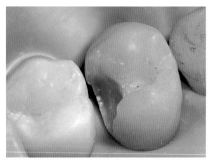

Fig 1-20 Prepared cavity on the distal and occlusal surfaces of an upper right first premolar tooth. The cavity is isolated with a rubber dam.

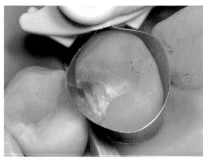

Fig 1-21 Metal matrix band held in place by interproximal wooden wedge.

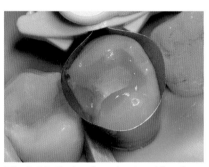

Fig 1-22 Orthophosphoric acid etchant being applied to the enamel and dentine of the prepared cavity. The etchant is then washed and lightly dried.

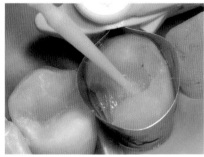

Fig 1-23 Enamel and dentine adhesive system being applied to the cavity with an applicator brush.

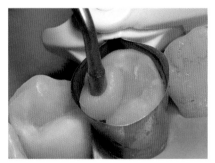

Fig 1-24 Placement of packable resin composite in the cavity using an amalgam packer.

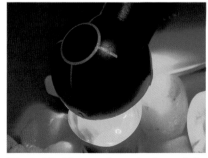

Fig 1-25 Photopolymerisation of the packable resin composite material.

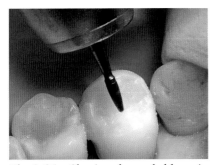

Fig 1-26 Shaping the packable resin composite, posterior restoration with tungsten carbide finishing burs. Water coolant is applied to avoid overheating of the restoration and tooth and to remove the grinding debris created.

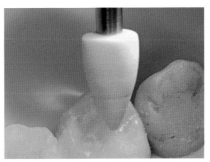

Fig 1-27 Polishing the packable resin composite with abrasive-impregnated rubber polishing point.

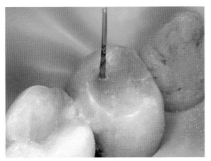

Fig 1-28 Etching the margins of the newly placed packable resin composite restoration with orthophosphoric acid. The etchant is then washed and lightly dried.

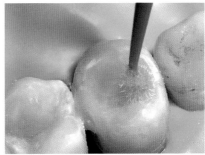

Fig 1-29 Sealant is applied to the surface of the resin composite restoration and then photopolymerised.

When posterior composites were first introduced, much research effort was expended on techniques to achieve tight proximal contacts to prevent food packing. This proved to be difficult, as early formulations not only lacked the viscosity to deform a matrix band under a packing force, but also would not hold a matrix tight against the adjacent tooth. The problem was compounded by the then popular use of clear plastic matrix bands, selected to allow multidirectional penetration of the curing light and increase polymerisation. These bands were too thick and, when removed, often left a light or missing contact with the adjacent tooth. In addition, they did not adapt well to the shape of the tooth. Subsequently, metal matrix systems have been shown to be more effective.

Whatever material is selected, great care must be taken when placing a posterior composite. Ideally, it should be placed under rubber dam to minimise the risk of a moisture-compromised bond between the restoration and the remaining tooth tissues.

Core Composites

Resin composites are increasingly used as a core build-up material in anterior and posterior teeth prior to placement of a full-coverage crown (Fig 1-30). Application is especially indicated in anterior teeth that are to be restored will all-ceramic crowns, where an aesthetic core material is required, notably in conjunction with a carbon or quartz fibre post. Core composites may be light-cured, to be applied in increments, or self-cure only, but more commonly they are dual-cured. Core composites are typically supplied as two pastes. A chemical-cure polymerisation reaction allows bulk placement, without concerns regarding penetration of the curing light to the depths of the preparation.

Core composites are often supplied in a shade that does not match the tooth substance. This ensures that when the crown preparation is carried out, it is easy to differentiate visually between the material and tooth tissue. This helps ensure that the margins are situated in dentine and not on the resin composite. This is important, as it is inadvisable to locate the crown margin coincident with, in particular, the composite–tooth junction, thereby minimising the potential for leakage and failure.

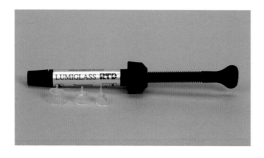

Fig 1-30 Syringe of resin composite designed for use as a core build-up material prior to placing a crown. Also shown are the clear plastic core-formers used to give the desired core geometry.

Resin composites have clinical advantages over amalgam in that they can be prepared for a crown at the same visit the core is placed and they contribute additional core retention through adhesive bonding. It is unwise, however, to depend solely on the adhesive properties of resin composite to resist the displacing forces applied to a crown or bridge. Extension of the crown margin apical to the composite–tooth junction will provide a protective ferrule effect, increasing retention and resistance. In cases in which most of the dentine has been lost, placement of additional mechanical retention features, such as a post (non-vital teeth) or possibly dentine pins (vital teeth), is prudent, in particular if insufficient dentine remains to accommodate retentive slots and groves.

However, resin composites have disadvantages as core materials compared with alternative materials such as amalgam. Resin composites deform plastically when subjected to cyclic loading, such as chewing, which may predispose to failure (Huysmans et al., 1992). In addition, composites expand when exposed to water, risking the possibility that the crown will not be an accurate fit.

Indirect Resin Composites
Indirect restorations such as crowns, veneers and inlays may be made from resin composite in the laboratory and then cemented in place using a composite luting cement. Laboratory production requires additional expense and clinical time recording impressions and making temporary restorations, but it gives the advantages of increased degree of polymerisation, wear resistance and density and enhanced mechanical properties. In addition, laboratory production permits increased control over proximal contacts and occlusal form. Restorations made in this manner may be subjected to increased light exposure, heat, pressure and vacuum to achieve certain advantages over resin composites cured directly in the mouth.

Ormocers
"Ormocer" is an acronym for "organically modified ceramic". It was a term created to describe a particular type of resin composite (Admira, Voco) recommended for anterior and posterior restorations, core build-up, splinting and veneers. Ormocers contain an inorganic–organic copolymer synthesised from multifunctional urethane and thioether(meth)acrylate alkoxysilanes. The filler particles are 1–1.5 µm, giving 61% filler by volume, or 77% by weight. Polymerisation contraction values as low as 1.97% have been reported.

Ceromers
"Ceromer" is another acronym created to describe a type of resin composite, standing for "ceramic optimised polymer" (Tetric Ceram, Ivoclar). Ceromers

contain barium glass fillers, spheroidal mixed oxide, ytterbium trifluoride and silicon dioxide. They exhibit all the properties of resin composite and release very small amounts of fluoride.

Fluoride-releasing Resin Composites

A small number of resin composites contain glass filler particles that release fluoride ions and have the ability to be *recharged* when exposed to external applications of fluoride. The level of fluoride release from most of these materials is, however, much lower than from compomers and from conventional and resin-modified glass ionomer cements. An exception to this (not available now) was an ion-releasing resin composite – Ariston pHc (Vivadent) – which released significant amounts of fluoride, hydroxyl and calcium ions as the pH adjacent to the restoration dropped when exposed to active demineralisation by plaque. This type of material was described as *smart* as it released ions to promote remineralisation and inhibit plaque growth, exactly when required. These materials are no longer commercially available as they demonstrated inferior physical properties, with high wear and reduced bond strength resulting in inferior clinical performance with increased incidence of tooth fracture and pulp hypersensitivity.

Advantages of Resin Composites

- Tooth-coloured, have excellent aesthetics and good colour stability.
- Mercury-free.
- Conservative of tooth substance as mechanical retention and resistance features are not required.
- Can be bonded to enamel and dentine.
- Low thermal conductivity, insulating pulp from temperature changes.
- No galvanic potential.

Disadvantages of Resin Composites

- Shrinkage on polymerisation (0.6–6% by volume); this creates stresses within the restored tooth unit, which can lead to cuspal flexure, cracking of enamel margins, breakdown of adhesive bond and propagation of hairline cracks in the remaining tooth tissue.
- The dentine–composite bond may degrade with time.
- The coefficient of thermal expansion of resin composite is typically two to six times higher than that of tooth substance. This leads to stress and potential breakdown of the adhesive bond between the restoration and the tooth.

- Working time is less than ideal for some materials due to premature polymerisation of resin composite under dental operating light.
- Sorption of water by resin composite. This can degrade the stability of the silane coupling between the resin matrix and the filler particles.
- Higher rate of secondary caries compared with amalgam or glass-ionomer restorations.
- Increased incidence of post-operative sensitivity compared with amalgam or glass-ionomer cement restorations.

Dimensional Stability

Polymerisation Shrinkage
Resin composites shrink on polymerisation, generating a significant stress within the material, which becomes more rigid as the set progresses. This contraction stress is constrained by the adhesive bond to the relatively rigid tooth structure. Initially, some relief of this stress is obtained by plastic deformation and flow of the resin composite, before it sets to a rigid mass. However, polymerisation proceeds very rapidly subsequent to photoinitiation, leaving little opportunity for stress relaxation to occur. The residual stress can cause:
- Deformation of the tooth cusps of up to 50 μm, which will predispose the tooth to cracked tooth syndrome. The deformation can also give rise to tooth sensitivity given deformation of the dentine tubules.
- Fracture of the enamel margins of the preparation.
- Failure of the adhesive bond to dentine. This may lead to leakage, marginal staining, secondary caries and pulpal inflammation.
- Damage to the structure of the resin composite.

Stresses can cause cracks to initiate within the restoration, especially at the filler–matrix interface. This occurs given the large difference between the elastic modulus (rigidity) of the filler particles and that of the matrix. The cracks can then propagate, ultimately causing bulk fracture of the restoration, when the internal stresses are suddenly released. The cracks propagate with additional stresses from thermal cycling (sudden changes in intraoral temperature during eating and drinking) and cyclic biting forces. Thermal cycling stresses the adhesive interface given the significantly higher coefficient of thermal expansion of the resin composite compared with the tooth structure. Thus, when exposed to hot substances, the resin composite expands more than the tooth, and when exposed to cold, it shrinks more than the tooth. This leads to cyclic stressing of the adhesive interface, especially at the dentine–restoration interface, with the potential to increase leakage. Microfill and flowable composites contain a relatively low volume of filler particles and therefore demonstrate high values of polymerisation contraction.

Incremental Packing Technique

The incremental packing technique advocates placing the resin composite in such a way as to minimise the surface area of each increment of resin composite bonded to tooth substance (Fig 1-31). This has the effect of maximising the surface area of resin composite that is free to shrink during polymerisation, relieving stress by plastic deformation. The resultant reduction in stress reduces the potential for adhesive breakdown, cuspal flexure, etc. Occlusal posterior resin composites generate the most stress as the entire periphery of resin composite is strongly restrained by the bond to enamel, while large multisurface restorations with proximal boxes or replacing missing cusps paradoxically generate less stress as they have larger surface areas which are free to shrink during polymerisation.

For many years it was believed that resin composites contracted towards the curing light, normally located over the occlusal surface of the preparation. This was thought to cause the resin composite to shrink away from the preparation, causing marginal gaps secondary to adhesive failure. Complex systems of clear plastic matrices and wedges were designed to allow curing light to be directed along the wedge to the first increment of resin composite on the gingival floor. Subsequent research has, however, shown that resin composite contracts towards the surface to which it is bonded (Versluis et al., 1998). Thus, adhesive bond failures along the gingival floor, which were very common with early resin composite restorations, may be attributable

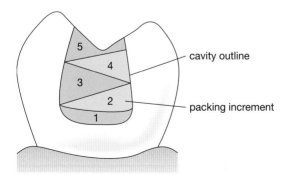

cavity outline

packing increment

Fig 1-31 The incremental packing technique, to help minimise polymerisation stresses.

to the relatively poor bond strengths of the older dentine adhesive systems and inadequate isolation, rather than to the light-curing technique.

The gingival margin of an occlusoproximal posterior composite is still the margin most likely to fail. Reasons for this failure include:

- Contamination of the gingival floor by saliva or blood in the absence of rubber dam isolation.
- There may only be dentine or dentine and cementum to bond to, which gives an inferior and less durable marginal bond than that to enamel.
- Difficulties in accessing the area to achieve optimal photopolymerisation.

The first increment of resin composite in a proximal box should be no more than 1 mm thick and carefully light-cured. Composites do not suffer adverse effects from extended light-curing. Subsequent increments of resin composite are placed obliquely in layers, ensuring that the resin contacts only the buccal or the lingual walls, but not both simultaneously. This helps minimise polymerisation stresses (Fig 1-31).

Uptake of Water
Over time, resin composites absorb water, leading to hygroscopic expansion. This counteracts the effects of polymerisation contraction to a small degree; however, it can take up to seven days for the expansion to match the polymerisation contraction. The damage caused by the shrinkage, outlined above, occurs in the first few seconds of light-curing. Once the cracks have initiated they cannot be healed by subsequent expansion. Microfill and flowable composites contain a reduced volume of filler particles and therefore demonstrate a higher uptake of water. Inadequately polymerised resin composites absorb more water than optimally polymerised composites.

The uptake of water can damage the structure of the resin composite. It has the potential to cause breakdown of the filler–matrix interface, leading to colour instability, reduced wear resistance and leaching of inorganic ions such as silicon, boron, barium and strontium. The release of ions increases the possibility of resin composite bioincompatibility.

Wear Resistance

Wear resistance is of particular significance for posterior resin composite restorations. Older formulations of resin composite wore excessively, causing significant clinical problems of passive eruption and marginal discrepancies. The wear of resin composite is related to the type, size and distribution of glass filler particles. Materials with less than 60% filler particles (by volume) demonstrate excessive wear when used to restore posterior teeth. Therefore, microfill and flowable composites are, in general, unsuitable for posterior use in load-bearing areas. Hybrid composites with larger mean particle sizes (>3 μm) show higher wear rates than those with smaller filler particles. This is a result of larger filler particles being "plucked" from the surface of the restoration when exposed to abrasive wear during mastication.

Wear rates will increase if there is an inadequate degree of polymerisation of the resin composite. This may occur if the light output (*irradiance*) of the dental curing light is too low, the curing tip is held too far from the surface of the restoration, the light is applied for too short a time period, or too thick an increment of resin composite is placed (see Chapter 8, page 111).

Wear is also related to the size of the restoration. Restorations that are wide and have a large surface area are more likely to include occlusal contact areas, resulting in increased wear compared with smaller restorations, where occlusal contact areas remain on unrestored enamel. Restorations in molar teeth tend to wear faster than those in premolars. This is thought to be related to the relatively higher biting forces applied to molars.

Resin composites are subjected to wear by mechanical abrasion and attrition, static and fatigue loads, and by chemical breakdown. Patients who clench or grind their teeth (bruxists) apply significantly higher loads to their teeth than non-bruxists. Normal chewing forces are around 35 N, while maximal clenching forces can be as high as 200 N on anterior teeth and 600 N on posterior teeth in adults.

The placement of posterior composite restorations in heavy bruxists is not advisable given the high risk of restoration failure by fracture and the possibility of cracked tooth syndrome. Under these circumstances, amalgam restorations will survive longer. Many clinical and laboratory-based studies have compared the wear characteristics of resin composites and dental amalgam restorations in posterior teeth. In general, posterior composites exhibit increased wear compared with amalgam, but smaller restorations of composite and amalgam show similar wear rates.

Survival of Posterior Composites

Posterior resin composite restorations are frequently chosen as an alternative to dental amalgam. To enable the patient and dentist to make an informed choice regarding which is appropriate, the longevity or probable survival of each type of material is relevant. Several studies have compared the survival of each material and have given differing results. Survival has been found to depend on the type of material used, the age and attendance pattern of the patient, the experience of the dentist and the clinical setting.

The vast majority of studies have shown that the survival and cost-effectiveness of dental amalgam is superior to resin composite for the restoration of posterior teeth (Chadwick et al., 2002). The placement of a resin composite restoration takes longer and is more technique-sensitive than an amalgam restoration, and this may explain why some studies have reported higher failure rates for posterior resin composites.

The reasons for failure of posterior resin composites are consistently reported as secondary caries and bulk fracture. Marginal breakdown, colour instability and postoperative sensitivity are less frequently reported.

References

Chadwick B, Dummer P, Dunstan F, et al. How long do fillings last? Evid Based Dent 2002;3:96–99.

Ferracane JL. Current trends in dental composites. Crit Rev Oral Biol Med 1995;6(4):302–318.

Huysmans MC, van der Varst PG, Schafer R, Peters MC, Plasschaert AJ, Soltesz U. Fatigue behavior of direct post-and-core-restored premolars. J Dent Res 1992;71(5): 1145–1150.

Powers JM, Sakaguchi RL (eds). Craig's Restorative Dental Materials. St Louis, Missouri: Mosby Elsevier, 2006.

Versluis A, Tantbirojn D, Douglas WH. Do dental composites always shrink toward the light? J Dent Res 1998;77(6):1435–1445.

Chapter 2
Compomers and Giomers

Aim

The aim of this chapter is to increase comprehension of compomers and giomers, including how they relate to other tooth-coloured, adhesive, restorative materials.

Outcome

Readers will become familiar with how the composition and physical properties of these newer materials differ from those of resin composites, together with their clinical indications and contraindications.

Compomers

Compomers are polyacid modified composite resins. These materials derive their name from merging parts of the descriptors "composite" and "glass-ionomer". The idea was to suggest that these new materials were a hybrid between composite resins and glass-ionomer cements, retaining the benefits of both while minimising their respective disadvantages. Thus, composite resins have superior strength, fracture toughness and aesthetics compared with glass-ionomer cements, but in general lack the ability to bond chemically to tooth substance and release fluoride. Compomers have been a successful addition to the range of direct restorative materials. Their popularity is largely attributed to their excellent, non-sticky handling. In appearance and performance, compomers are more closely related to composite resins than glass-ionomer cements. Trends in material properties for resin composites, compomers, conventional and resin-modified glass-ionomer cements are set out in Fig 2-1.

Indications

Compomers are recommended by manufacturers for the restoration of:
• all types of cavities in deciduous teeth
• cervical cavities (carious or non-carious) in adults
• anterior proximal restorations in adults

- small load–bearing restorations in adults,

and also:

- as a temporary or transitional restorative material
- as a core build–up material if at least 50% of coronal dentine is still available.

In addition, one compomer (Dyract AP, Dentsply) is recommended by the manufacturer for the restoration of all types of cavities in children and adults, including stress–bearing occlusal surfaces, where the cavity is less than two–thirds the intercuspal distance.

The presentation of a compomer material is shown in Fig 2-2. The clinical placement of a compomer material in a cervical cavity in an upper left central incisor tooth is illustrated in Figs 2-3 to 2-9.

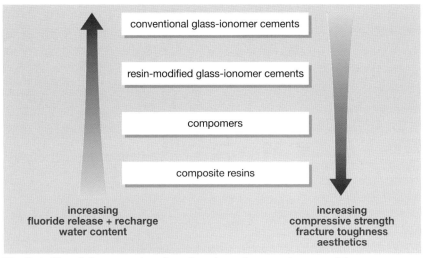

Fig 2-1 Trends in properties of tooth–coloured restorative materials.

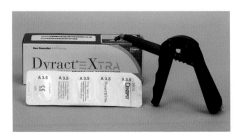

Fig 2-2 A compomer restorative material, showing the compule and applicator gun.

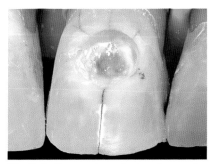

Fig 2-3 Prepared cervical cavity on the labial aspect of an upper left central incisor tooth.

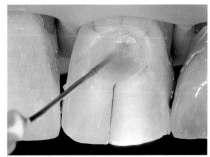

Fig 2-4 Orthophosphoric acid etchant being applied to the enamel and dentine of the prepared cavity. The etchant is then washed and lightly dried.

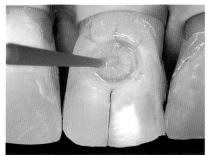

Fig 2-5 Enamel and dentine adhesive system being applied to the cavity with an applicator brush.

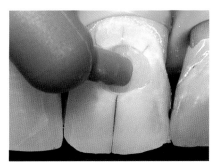

Fig 2-6 Placement of compomer in the cavity.

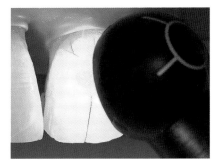

Fig 2-7 Photopolymerisation of the compomer restoration.

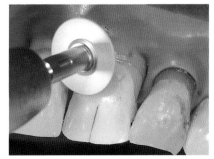

Fig 2-8 Polishing the compomer with small-diameter aluminium oxide abrasive discs.

25

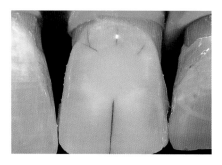

Fig 2-9 The finished compomer restoration.

Contraindications

Compomers have been contraindicated in the following clinical situations:
- where a direct or indirect pulp cap is required
- a core build-up for an all-ceramic crown
- where a dry field cannot be achieved
- where the patient has an allergy to dimethacrylate resins
- where the restoration will be in contact with a eugenol-containing lining or base material, which will interfere with the polymerisation of the compomer.

Composition

Compomers are resin-based materials but their composition varies between brands. In general, compomers contain:
- polymerisable resins with methacrylate and polycarboxylate groups
- glass filler particles, such as fluoroaluminosilicate, strontium fluorosilicate or barium fluorosilicate glass
- photoinitiators (camphorquinone/amine system)
- stabilisers.

The polymerisable resins of some commercially available compomers contain significantly more carboxylate groups than other compomers, which contain more methacrylate groups. Materials with methacrylate groups behave predominantly like composite resins. Those with a high proportion of carboxylate groups behave more like glass-ionomer cements. The first commercially available compomer (Dyract, Dentsply) contained the polymerisable resins urethane dimethacrylate (UDMA) and TCB resin, an acid monomer – a bi-ester of 2-hydroxyethyl methacrylate (2-HEMA) and butane tetracarboxylic acid – which contained both carboxylate and methacrylate groups.

Initially, the filler particles were strontium fluorosilicate glass with a mean particle size of 2.5 μm and 70% filler loading by weight (47% by volume). Thus, this compomer contained the components of glass-ionomer cement – acidic polycarboxylate groups and basic strontium fluoroaluminosilicate glass (see Chapter 4, pages 53-54) together with the methacrylate groups that undergo light-activated free radical polymerisation, as occurs with most composite resins (see Chapter 1, pages 3–4) (Burke et al., 2002).

This material has been replaced by a newer version (Dyract AP, Dentsply), which has a similar chemistry but has been modified by the addition of smaller glass filler particles (0.8 μm) and a new, more highly cross-linked monomer. These changes are stated by the manufacturer to give the material increased strength, fracture toughness, wear resistance and fluoride release and improved polishability.

An alternative compomer material (F2000, 3M ESPE) contains the polymerisable resin CDMA, a dimethacrylate functional oligomer derived from citric acid, which acts as the acidic hydrophilic matrix former, and glyceryl dimethacrylate (GDMA), which acts as a hydrophilic co-monomer and CDMA diluent. An additional high molecular weight, hydrophilic polymer is added to modify material handling properties and aid the transport of water and fluoride in the compomer. This compomer contains 3–10 μm fluoroaluminosilicate glass filler particles (84% filler by weight).

Hytac (3M ESPE) contains the polymerisable resins methacrylated phosphoric acid ester (MPAE) and UDMA. This compomer contains zinc-calcium-alumino-fluoro-silicate glass and ytterbium trifluoride glass fillers (81% filler by weight) of average particle size 5 μm.

The compomer Compoglass F (Ivoclar Vivadent) contains the polymerisable resins UDMA, tetraethylene glycol dimethacrylate and cycloaliphatic dicarboxylic acid dimethacrylate (DCDMA). The glass filler particles are barium aluminofluorosilicate glass, ytterbium trifluoride and spheroid mixed oxides. The particle size is 0.2–3.0 μm, 55% filler by volume (77% by weight).

Setting Reaction

- Compomer is exposed to a curing light and the free radical polymerisation reaction is initiated by a camphorquinone/amine system.
- The polymerisable resin molecules intermingle to become a resin matrix reinforced with glass filler particles.

- Later, when exposed to saliva in the mouth, water is absorbed by the matrix over a period of days and weeks, and permits the acidic polycarboxylate groups and basic glass filler particles to react, creating further ionic cross-linking of the matrix and release of small amounts of fluoride (Burke et al., 2002).

Fluoride Release

Compomers are part of a spectrum of materials that release fluoride (Fig 2-1). Fluoride release is related to water content, and in general there is an inverse relationship between fluoride release and physical properties. The ability to release fluoride is considered beneficial because it has the potential to help prevent dental caries. This effect is thought to act in several ways (Featherstone, 2000), whereby fluoride:

- diffuses into cariogenic bacteria and inhibits bacterial metabolism by altering enzyme activity
- inhibits demineralisation when present at the enamel crystal surface during an acid challenge from bacteria
- enhances remineralisation of enamel by formation of a low-solubility crystal veneer similar to fluorapatite.

The interaction between fluoride from restorative materials and secondary caries adjacent to the margins of restorations is complex. The initial high burst of fluoride release in the first hours after the placement of a fluoride-releasing material is short-lived, and speculation therefore remains as to whether the material can help prevent secondary caries in the months and years after placement. A systematic review of the published literature found that there was no conclusive evidence for or against a treatment effect of inhibition of secondary caries by glass-ionomer cements (Randall and Wilson, 1999).

A significant factor in the ability of a material to help prevent caries in the longer term is the ability to replace, or *recharge*, the fluoride within the material for continued slow-release. This new fluoride is obtained in the oral environment from applied fluoride-containing toothpastes, mouthrinses, gels or varnishes. The recharging ability of glass-ionomer cements is higher than that of compomers, which in turn is higher than that of composite resin. Following recharge, compomer demonstrates a burst of fluoride release for one day, which returns to baseline levels after two to three days (Xu and Burgess, 2003).

A significant factor affecting the ability of the material to recharge with fluoride is thought to be the structure of the hydrogel layer around the glass filler particles, following the reaction between the glass and the polyacid. Glass-ionomer cements demonstrate an extensive hydrogel layer, while compomers have a limited layer, due to the constraints placed on the acid–base setting reaction occurring in the days after the main polymerisation reaction of the resin components. The fluoride is released during formation of the hydrogel layer, and it is suggested that the fluoride taken up during recharging occupies the sites previously occupied by fluoride, prior to its release.

Fluoride is released when the acid–base setting reaction described above is initiated by water absorption in the first few days and weeks in the mouth. Compomers give an early low burst of fluoride, less than 10 mg/cm^2 per day, but this is sustained for a relatively long time. The release of fluoride is increased when the size of the fluoride-containing glass filler particle reduces. Manufacturers have made use of this fact and reduced particle size when producing newer, improved versions of their products.

Physical Properties

Compomers have slightly lower compressive, diametral tensile and flexural strengths than hybrid composite resins. In addition, they demonstrate reduced fracture toughness and hardness, reflected clinically in higher wear rates. Conversely, the physical properties of compomers tend to be better than those of resin-modified glass-ionomer cements, which in turn are in general better than those of conventional glass-ionomer cements.

Bond to Tooth Substance

Hypothetically, compomers have the potential to bond to tooth substance by two mechanisms. First, a chemical bond – through the methacrylate groups – to the dentine adhesive micromechanically retained to dentine and enamel, in the same manner that composite resins bond to tooth (see Chapter 3, pages 39-41). Second, the acid–base glass-ionomer components could potentially create an ionic bond to tooth substance (see Chapter 4, pages 63-64). However, compomers require the application of a bonding agent to bond to tooth substance, and they do not cure without exposure to light. As a consequence, the inherent bond to enamel and dentine displayed by glass-ionomer cements would appear to be absent.

Each compomer manufacturer advises use of its own bonding agent to bond the material to the tooth. Most adhesives are self-etching, and thus the penetration into the dentine is much less than when an etch-and-rinse technique with phosphoric acid is used (see Chapter 3, pages 41-44). Similarly, the acid is insufficiently aggressive to create a highly retentive etch pattern on enamel. The bond strength of compomers to dentine and enamel is slightly lower when a self-etch adhesive is used (21 MPa to dentine, 19 MPa to enamel) compared with an etch-and-rinse technique (22 MPa to dentine, 23 MPa to enamel), and both are lower than the bond strength of composite resins to dentine and enamel. This is reflected in a reduction in marginal integrity of compomer restorations compared with composite restorations. Marginal integrity can be improved when bonding compomer to enamel by the use of an etch-and-rinse bonding agent, rather than use of the self-etch adhesive supplied.

Dimensional Stability

Compomers undergo polymerisation shrinkage in the same manner as composite resins. This is followed by a slow absorption of water (hygroscopic expansion), which may result in a small net linear expansion over a period of several weeks. This hygroscopic expansion is significantly higher in compomers than in composite resins and may help to offset the relatively larger marginal gaps seen around compomer restorations, when compared with composite restorations, at initial placement. The clinical significance of marginal gaps is discussed in Chapter 6 (pages 88-89).

Giomers

Giomer is a term given to a small number of materials (made by one manufacturer, Shofu Inc.), which, like compomers, were developed in an attempt to retain the clinical advantages of glass–ionomer cements while minimising their disadvantages, specifically their poorer aesthetics and vulnerability to dehydration. Giomers are resin-based materials containing urethane dimethacrylate and hydroxyethyl methacrylate, with the addition of prereacted glass–ionomer particles (PRG). The particles are similar to the fluorosilicate glasses found in glass–ionomer cements. They are reacted with polyacrylic acid prior to addition to the resin. The prereaction can involve either the surface of the particles (Beautifil) or almost the entire particle (Reactmer). Giomers set by photopolymerisation are highly radiopaque, and they require a bonding agent to bond to tooth substance.

The manufacturer of giomers recommends their use in the following situations:

- all types of cavities in deciduous teeth
- all types of cavities in adult teeth
- core build-ups
- the repair of composite and porcelain restorations.

Early research gave conflicting results regarding the ability of giomers to release fluoride. One study (Itota et al., 2004) reported that a full-reaction-type prereacted giomer (Reactmer, Shofu Inc.) released significantly more fluoride than a compomer and a composite resin, and, in addition, it re-released the greatest amount of fluoride following the fluoride recharge. In contrast, another study (Yap et al., 2002) found that the giomer did not have an initial burst of fluoride release, and that although fluoride release was high in the short term, at 28 days it was lower than from a compomer.

The surface roughness of giomers following finishing and polishing with aluminium oxide discs was comparable with that of compomer and composite resin and, therefore, significantly smoother than glass-ionomer cement. Further research into the dimensional stability of giomers is required given the extent to which these materials absorb water. In addition, further clinical studies are required to better understand the clinical performance of these materials and to determine if they warrant recognition as a distinctly new restorative material.

References

Burke FJ, Fleming GJ, Owen FJ, Watson DJ. Materials for restoration of primary teeth: 2. Glass ionomer derivatives and compomers. Dent Update 2002;29(1):10–14.

Featherstone JD. The science and practice of caries prevention. J Am Dent Assoc 2000;131(7):887–899.

Itota T, Carrick TE, Yoshiyama M, McCabe JF. Fluoride release and recharge in giomer, compomer and resin composite. Dent Mater J, 2004;20(9):789–795.

Randall RC, Wilson NHF. Glass-ionomer restoratives: a systematic review of a secondary caries treatment effect. J Dent Res 1999;78(2):628–637.

Xu X, Burgess JO. Compressive strength, fluoride release and recharge of fluoride-releasing materials. Biomaterials 2003;24(14):2451–2461.

Yap AU, Tham SY, Zhu LY, Lee HK. Short term fluoride release from various aesthetic restorative materials. Oper Dent 2002;27(3):259–265.

Chapter 3
Enamel and Dentine Adhesive Systems

Aim

The aim of this chapter is to provide an update on the confusing array of enamel and dentine adhesive systems available for clinical use with restorative materials.

Outcome

Readers will understand the mode of action of the bond between enamel and dentine adhesive systems and dental substrates. This understanding will aid comprehension of the advantages and disadvantages of each system, including bond durability.

Introduction

Adhesive dentistry is widely considered to have begun when Buonocore described in 1955 a method of bonding acrylic filling materials to enamel by the application of acid to the enamel as a surface pretreatment. In 1968 Buonocore hypothesised that the bond was based on the creation of resin tags engaging microporosities in acid-etched enamel (Buonocore et al., 1968).

The Structure of Enamel

Enamel consists (by volume) of 86% inorganic hydroxyapatite crystals, 12% water and 2% organic matrix (Fig 3-1). The hydroxyapatite crystals, which are the shape of flattened hexagons, are tightly packed together in the shape of prisms and bound together by the organic matrix. The crystals are not "pure" hydroxyapatite $(Ca^{10}(PO_4)^6(OH)_2)$ but have carbonate molecules substituted within the lattice. This is deleterious to the acid resistance of enamel, as the carbonate groups are more susceptible to demineralisation. Fortunately, however, fluoride ions can also be substituted into the lattice network, forming fluoroapatite or fluorohydroxyapatite, which is more resistant to demineralisation. These fluoride ions can be obtained by topical application of fluoride-containing toothpastes, mouthrinses or varnishes, or released by fluoride-releasing dental restorative materials.

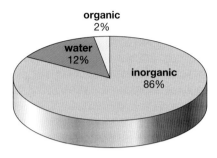

Fig 3-1 Composition of human enamel.

The crystals are bound together to form enamel *prisms*. A network of interconnecting spaces and micropores exists between the crystals, which provides a pathway for the diffusion of fluids, ions and other low molecular weight substances between the oral environment, the dentinal tubules and, ultimately, the pulp. Therefore, topical applications of agents such as fluoride or bleaching agents are not only active on the surface of the tooth, but also have the potential to diffuse through the full thickness of enamel.

Bonding to Enamel

Restorative materials can be bonded to the surface of enamel by the topical application of acid. The most commonly used acid is orthophosphoric acid, which, when applied to enamel for around 15 s, removes around 10 μm of the surface, prior to creating a range of etch patterns, which may involve loss of enamel prism periphery, loss of enamel prism core or a diffuse appearance with no specific pattern.

This surface etching increases the surface area of enamel hugely and creates pores, up to 20 μm deep, that become filled on contact with restorative materials. Etching also raises the surface energy of enamel and increases the ability of applied bonding resins to wet the surface, ensuring intimate adaptation. A low-viscosity hydrophobic bonding resin is then applied, which will often contain bis-GMA, UDMA, HEMA or TEGDMA. Photopolymerisation (light-curing) of the bonding resin creates micromechanical retention between the enamel and the resin. Bonding resins bond chemically with the methacrylate groups of subsequently applied restorative material by copolymerisation. The clinical use of etchant and enamel and dentine adhesive systems is illustrated in Figs 1-15, 1-16, 2-4 and 2-5.

The optimum concentration of phosphoric acid is around 37%. Higher concentrations cause precipitation of salts that inhibit further demineralisation of the enamel. It is important to adequately wash away the demineralised enamel components for 5–10 s and to dry the enamel with compressed air from a three-in-one syringe. Care must be taken not to dry any exposed dentine excessively as this may reduce the bond strength to dentine and cause post-operative sensitivity. When correctly applied, reliable and durable bond strengths of 20 MPa are obtained. This bond strength can be greatly reduced if the enamel is contaminated with blood or saliva during the bonding process. It is therefore important to maintain a clean, dry field by isolating the tooth, ideally with a rubber dam. The bond to dentine is less reliable and subject to breakdown over time; therefore, restorations bonded to enamel around all of the cavity periphery are less likely to experience failure of the adhesive bond compared with restorations bonded at least in part to margins of dentine.

The Structure of Dentine

Human dentine consists of 50% (by volume) mineral, which is a carbonate-rich and calcium-deficient apatite, 30% organic material, largely Type I collagen, and 20% dentinal fluid (Fig 3-2). It also contains very small amounts of other proteins and organic components (Marshall et al., 1997).

Dentine comprises tubules containing odontoblast processes and fluid, with the numbers increasing from the enamel–dentine junction towards the pulp chamber. The tubule lumen is lined by highly mineralised peritubular dentine with apatite crystals and some organic matrix. The tubules are separated by intertubular dentine, which is less mineralised and contains a matrix of Type I collagen reinforced with apatite. Dentinal tubules are more numerous and

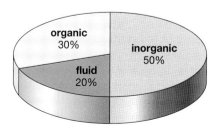

Fig 3-2 Composition of human dentine.

have a larger diameter close to the pulp. The tubules gradually become smaller in diameter and less numerous towards the enamel–dentine junction. Dentinal fluid is under a slight positive pressure from the pulp (25–30 mmHg). The clinical significance of this is that cavities that cut into deep dentine have a larger proportion of cut tubules exuding wet dentinal fluid than superficial cavities.

There are many different types of dentine: primary and secondary, formed physiologically; and tertiary – sclerotic, transparent, carious, demineralised, remineralised and hypermineralised – altered by age and disease processes (Marshall et al., 1997). These variations in dentine morphology result in bonds with adhesive restorative systems being variable.

Non-carious cervical lesions are difficult defects in which to retain a composite resin restoration with a dentine adhesive system. These lesions are formed by combinations of erosion, abrasion and abfraction. The dentine tubules are occluded by mineral deposits with hypermineralisation of the intertubular dentine. The peritubular and intertubular dentine is more resistant to demineralisation and, as a consequence, the hybrid layer is much thinner and with few, if any, tubule resin tags.

Bonding to Dentine

Cavity Preparation and Smear Layer
Dental instrumentation produces a smear layer which covers the underlying dentine structure and penetrates several microns into the dentinal tubules, forming smear plugs. The smear layer, which is typically 0.5–5.0 μm thick, is easily dissolved in weak acids. It consists of partially denatured collagen and mineral, sometimes bacteria, and is only weakly adherent to the underlying dentine, with a bond strength of up to 5 MPa (Pashley, 1992). Early generations of dentine adhesive systems attempted to bond to the smear layer, but given its inherent weakness, unacceptably low bond strengths were obtained.

Types of Acid Etchants
Phosphoric acid is the most commonly used acid etchant; however, nitric, citric and maleic acids are also sometimes used. Most recent formulations of etchants are in the form of a gel, rather than a liquid, as gels are easier to place and control. Gels are formed by the addition of silica particles or polymer thickening agents to a liquid. Concerns have been expressed as to whether gels containing silica leave a residue of particles that may interfere with bonding, but this does not appear to be the case, let alone clinically significant.

Types of Dentine Adhesive Systems

Dentine adhesive systems can be classified according to either their order of introduction to clinical practice – first, second, third, fourth, fifth, sixth and seventh generation – or by a description of their action. Classification by action will be used here to aid understanding of clinical applications.

Etch-and-rinse Adhesives

These dentine adhesive systems require the application of an acid etchant or conditioner to the surface of the dentine. After a prescribed time, the etchant is washed away and the dentine dried with compressed air. This is followed by the application of a primer and then the adhesive resin. In three-step systems the primer and adhesive are applied sequentially, and in two-step systems the primer and adhesive are combined into one bottle. Examples of three-step and two-step etch-and-rinse adhesives are illustrated in Figs 3-3 and 3-4.

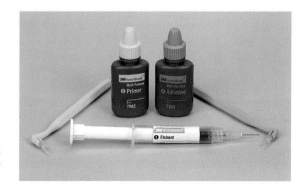

Fig 3-3 Example of a three-step etch-and-rinse adhesive system.

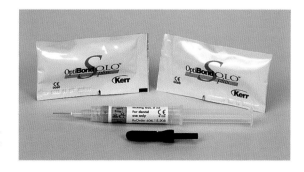

Fig 3-4 Example of a two-step etch-and-rinse adhesive system.

Etchants and Conditioners

Acids applied to tooth structure to demineralise enamel and dentine are referred to as etchants or conditioners. Their effect on enamel is described on page 34, and when applied to dentine they demineralise the surface, exposing collagen fibrils, which intermingle with the applied adhesive to form the *hybrid layer*, first described by Nakabayashi et al. in 1982. The conditioner is usually 30–40% orthophosphoric acid, but may be nitric, citric or maleic acid, and is usually applied to dentine at the same time, or slightly after, it is applied to any adjacent enamel.

The network of collagen fibrils formed by etching is susceptible to collapse if the fibrils become dehydrated. If it is in a collapsed state, the adhesive resin cannot adequately intermingle with it and produce a hybrid layer. Collapse occurs if the drying of the dentine after rinsing away the etchant is too prolonged or vigorous. Collapse of the network can, however, be reversed by rehydrating the collagen by application of a water-based primer. Water-free primers cannot rehydrate collagen and if applied to overdry dentine are ineffective in helping to create a hybrid layer. An alternative approach is "wet bonding", in which the ideal degree of hydration of the dentine is described as a shiny moist surface. Excess pools of water should be removed by blotting with a pledget or a sponge applicator brush, as its presence dilutes the primer, reducing its effectiveness.

When wet bonding, the primer often contains volatile solvents such as ethanol or acetone which seek out water and displace it. These volatile solvents are evaporated by application of a gentle stream of compressed air. The risk exists that if not all the water inside the collagen network is adequately displaced, phase separation of hydrophobic and hydrophilic components can occur, resulting in the formation of "blisters" at the resin–dentine interface. These disrupt the adhesive bond. Wet bonding is therefore very technique-sensitive, as both overdry and overwet conditions are undesirable.

Additional difficulties include the inability to visually assess adjacent enamel for a frosted appearance, indicating an adequate etch, and the tendency for volatile components to evaporate from the primer bottle during use. After an unpredictable period of time, the quantity of ethanol or acetone in the primer may be too low to adequately displace water and facilitate adhesive resin to infiltrate into the hybrid layer.

An alternative approach is the use of water-based primers (Adper Scotchbond Multipurpose, 3M ESPE; OptiBond, Kerr) which have the ability to rehydrate overdry collagen, and also displace excess water from dentine, as may be required. These adhesives are thought to be less technique-sensitive, giving a more reliable bond to dentine. The use of a dry bonding technique permits visual inspection for frosted enamel.

Primers

Primers are hydrophilic monomers that may be dissolved in a variety of solvents, including alcohol, acetone or water. Application of an acid etchant leaves the dentine with a relatively low surface energy, making it difficult for the adhesive to effectively wet the surface and infiltrate the collagen network to produce the hybrid layer. The role of a primer is to act as a wetting agent, infiltrating the hydrophilic surface of the etched dentine and collagen fibrils and displacing any water present. Separately applied primers are often lightly air-dried to aid evaporation of the solvent and expedite removal of water. Overenthusiastic air-drying can blast the primer off the surface, resulting in incomplete coverage of the dentine. A complete, shiny layer is a prerequisite to converting the hydrophilic dentine into a more hydrophobic environment, allowing infiltration of the hydrophobic adhesive (Nakabayashi and Takarada, 1992). Thus the primer is a bifunctional monomer that can form a bond between the hydrophilic collagen fibrils and the hydrophobic adhesive resin. HEMA is frequently present in primers given its excellent ability to wet enamel and dentine. Other monomers used include dipentaerythritol penta acrylate monophosphate (PENTA) and biphenyl dimethacrylate (BPDM).

Bonding Resin

The bonding resin usually consists of hydrophobic monomers such as bis-GMA, UDMA and TEGDMA, sometimes with HEMA added to increase hydrophilicity. The resin diffuses into the collagen network created by the application of the etchant and primer. On polymerisation the resin stabilises the hybrid layer, and where it has flowed into the exposed dentinal tubules, resin tags are formed.

The polymerisation can be light-activated as a separate step, prior to application of the restorative material, light-activated with the overlying restorative material, chemically activated or, light- and chemically activated, described as "dual-cured". It is thought beneficial to photopolymerise the adhesive resin as a separate step as this ensures adequate exposure to light, giving optimum polymerisation and applying the lowest disruptive stress to the newly forming adhesive bond. If the adhesive bond and restorative material are photopolymerised in one step, the risk exists that inadequate amounts of light will reach the adhesive, leading to sub-optimum polymerisation. This can increase the risk of degradation of the adhesive bond by hydrolysis and also increase the release of uncured monomer, with the potential for allergic or other systemic reactions. In addition, the overlying restorative material will be undergoing polymerisation contraction (see Chapter 1, page 4), which has the potential to significantly disrupt the bond of the adhesive resin to dentine, in particular, if the bond has been compromised. Chemically cured and dual-cured adhesives have the advantage of autopolymerisation even in conditions of sub-optimum light exposure.

Initially it was thought that resin tags were largely responsible for resin bonding to dentine. Subsequent research has shown that the hybrid layer is complex. Resin flows into the walls of tubules, creating tubule wall hybridisation, lateral branches off the main tubules, and intermingles with demineralised intertubular dentine. The structure of the dentine–adhesive interface where etchant and adhesive have been applied and following placement and photopolymerisation of a resin composite is depicted in Fig 3-5.

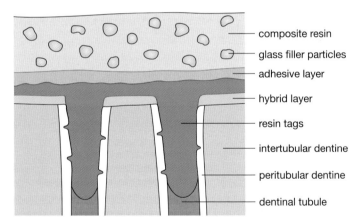

composite resin

glass filler particles

adhesive layer

hybrid layer

resin tags

intertubular dentine

peritubular dentine

dentinal tubule

Fig 3-5 The structure of the interface between adhesive and dentine, to which etchant and adhesive have been applied, following placement and photopolymerisation of a resin composite. This pattern of bond, with deep resin tags, is found in three-step etch-and-rinse adhesives, two-step etch-and-rinse adhesives and strong (low pH) self-etch adhesives. The smear layer has been removed and resin tags are present within the dentinal tubules, giving micromechanical retention. The adhesive combines with the surface demineralised dentine to form the hybrid layer.

The clinical advantages of etch-and-rinse adhesives include:
- a high and reliable bond strength to enamel
- long-term clinical data confirming clinical effectiveness
- versatility for bonding any type of restoration.

Three-step etch-and-rinse adhesives are considered by many to be the "gold standard", against which all other adhesives should be compared, as they are less technique-sensitive and give higher bond strengths to both enamel and dentine. Significant developments have occurred since such adhesives were first introduced, reducing the number of clinical steps and the time required to create a bond; however, these have been at the expense of the strength of the bond to enamel or the durability of the bond to dentine.

Stripping back the smear layer increases the permeability of the dentine by up to 90%. This may result in a high level of post-operative sensitivity. This is thought to be related to the aggressive etching action of the phosphoric acid opening up dentinal tubules which may subsequently not all be sealed by the adhesive. Three-step etch-and-rinse materials have, however, an established track record of clinical efficacy. The small increase in time required to place them compared with one- and two-step adhesives is fully justified if the performance and survival of the restoration are enhanced. Faster is not necessarily better.

With two-step etch-and-rinse adhesives where the primer and adhesive are combined in one bottle the small saving in clinical time is countered by a number of disadvantages, including inferior bonding to dentine and relatively poor marginal adaptation and durability.

Self-etch Adhesives

These adhesives do not require the application of an acid etchant or conditioner to the surface of the dentine. The adhesive contains carboxylic or phosphate acidic monomers (MDP, phenyl-P, MAC-10), which simultaneously condition and prime the dentine, together with cross-linking monomers (bis-GMA, UDMA, HEMA, TEGDMA) and solvent, often water. In two-step self-etch systems, the conditioner and primer are typically combined in one bottle, with the adhesive in a second. In the most recent one-step self-etch systems, the conditioner, primer and adhesive are all combined in one bottle. Self-etch adhesives do not require the rinsing and air-drying steps. The adhesive is spread by means of compressed air. Examples of one-step self-etch systems are shown in Figs 3-6 to 3-8.

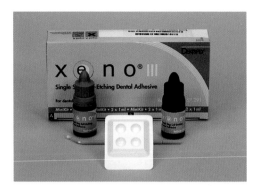

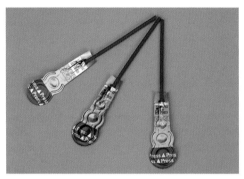

Figs 3-6 and **3-7**
Examples of one-step self-etch adhesive systems.

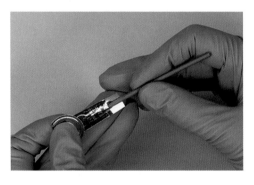

Fig 3-8 Example of a one-step self-etch adhesive system being activated by bending over the foil package and squeezing between the fingers.

Self-etch adhesives were developed in an attempt to improve clinical performance by:
- eliminating variables in rinsing
- reducing technique sensitivity through the elimination of the need to judge how wet or dry the dentine is after washing away a conditioner

- reducing the likelihood that dentine tubules would be opened up by application of a conditioner and then not fully occluded with the adhesive, which leads to post-operative sensitivity.

Self-etch adhesives do, however, have potential disadvantages:
- Those with a less acidic pH (milder etching capacity) do not etch uncut aprismatic enamel well, limiting subsurface demineralisation and resin tag formation. This can lead to relatively low bond strengths and unaesthetic staining of enamel margins (Tay and Pashley, 2003). This effect can be minimised by pre-etching the enamel with phosphoric acid; however, it is important that the phosphoric acid does not come into contact with any adjacent dentine as it will compromise the hybrid layer and reduce the bond strength to dentine.
- Short clinical track record.
- Lower bond strengths to dentine compared with three-step etch-and-rinse adhesives.
- Many adhesives require storage in a refrigerator.

Self-etch adhesives have been classified as *mild*, *intermediary strong* or *strong*, depending on their pH. Self-etch adhesives described as mild have a pH of around 2. These adhesives do not completely remove the smear layer, causing only superficial, incomplete demineralisation (1 µm deep) of the dentine. As a consequence, limited microporosities are created, resulting in a thin submicron hybrid layer. As the smear layer is not completely removed, resin tags are not formed. The retention of some hydroxyapatite crystals within the dentine gives the potential for chemical bonding to carboxylic acid and phosphate-based monomers. Bond strengths to enamel with mild self-etch adhesives are low; however, the bond to dentine appears clinically adequate. The advantage claimed for these materials is the superior long-term durability of the bond, due to the calcium–carboxylate and calcium–phosphate bonds and the ability to increase resistance to bond degradation through the hydrolysis of collagen.

Strong self-etch adhesives have low pH (<1) and their effect on dentine is similar to that seen with etch-and-rinse adhesives (Fig 3-5) extensive demineralisation, creation of a 4 µm-thick hybrid layer, resin tags extending into the dentinal tubules and laterally into the tubule walls. Retention is based on infiltration of the exposed collagen network and underlying dentine by the adhesive resin, with few opportunities for chemical interaction between acidic groups and hydroxyapatite crystals. Strong self-etch adhesives achieve good bond strengths to enamel but weaker bonds to dentine, compared with mild adhesives. It has been reported that residual water remains within the hybrid layer and cannot be removed, compromising the bond strength (De Munck et al., 2005b).

Some self-etch adhesives have a pH around 1.5, creating a different etch pattern. These adhesives are called "intermediary strong" adhesives. As the name suggests, these adhesives completely demineralise the surface of the hybrid layer and partially demineralise the base. There is a gradual transition between the hybrid layer and the underlying dentine. The effects of the acid component of an intermediary strong self-etch adhesive on the structure of dentine are shown in Fig 3-9a. The nature of the adhesive bond between the composite resin and the dentine is depicted in Fig 3-9b. These intermediary adhesives create a deeper etch pattern in both enamel and dentine compared with mild adhesives. Larger amounts of hydroxyapatite are available for potential chemical bonding to acidic groups of the adhesive than with the strong adhesives. Further research is required on all of these relatively new self-etch adhesives to determine if the intermediary strong adhesives give the optimum combination of enamel and dentine bonding or an unsatisfactory compromise of both.

Potential Problems with One-step Self-etch Adhesives

- There is a weak bond to enamel if a self-etch adhesive is not protected by the placement of an overlying composite restoration. This may occur with fissure sealing or using resin to treat dentine sensitivity. When unprotected by composite, the adhesive bond suffers osmotic blistering. In this process the resin acts as a permeable membrane, allowing water from the external environment, attracted by the hydrophilic and acidic resin monomers, to move through it. The blistering ultimately causes delamination of the resin.

- A similar process of water movement is described when one-step self-etch adhesives are bonded to hydrated dentine, leading to the phenomenon of "water trees". Water trees are interconnecting water-filled channels visible under transmission electron microscopy. These water-filled channels permit further water movement through the hybrid and adhesive layers, leading to formation of water blisters at the adhesive–composite interface. These blisters weaken the adhesive bond to dentine and may accelerate degradation of the bond over time.

- One-step, self-etch adhesives may be incompatible with chemically or dual-cured composites. When certain chemically or dual-cured composite resins

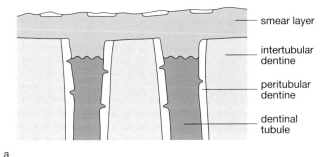

smear layer

intertubular dentine

peritubular dentine

dentinal tubule

a

composite resin

glass filler particles

adhesive resin impregnated smear layer

shallow resin tag

intertubular dentine

peritubular dentine

dentinal tubule

b

Figs 3-9 (a) The effects of the acid component of an intermediary strong self-etch adhesive on the structure of dentine. The upper part of the smear layer is completely demineralised and the lower part is partially demineralised. (b) The nature of the adhesive bond after application of the composite resin to the prepared dentine. An adhesive resin impregnated smear layer is produced, together with short resin tags extending into the dentinal tubules.

are placed over one-step self-etch adhesives there is a high risk of the restoration debonding. This may occur when a chemically cured composite is placed in bulk as a core build-up material, or when a dual-cured resin-based luting cement is used to bond indirect restorations, including crowns and posts. This problem occurs because chemically cured composites usually contain basic (alkaline) tertiary amines as catalysts. These amines react with the uncured acidic resin monomers of the surface oxygen-inhibited layer of the adhesive. This acid–base incompatibility can be rectified by mixing one-step self-etch adhesive with a separate bottle of a chemical co-initiator containing sodium benzene sulphinate. Thus, manufacturers supply an additional bottle with these systems, recommending its use when bonding dual-cured composite and luting cements. Some of the recent one-step self-etch adhesives include co-initiators within their formulation to overcome this problem. However, when using a dual-cured composite resin or luting cement it is prudent to use a three-step etch-and-rinse system or a two-step self-etch system to overcome the potential problem.

The problem does not occur with three-step etch-and-rinse adhesives or two-step self-etch adhesives as they are covered by a layer of neutral adhesive. This layer separates the acidic monomers from the basic amines of the self-cured composite.

- Chemically cured composites pose an additional problem for one-step self-etch adhesives. The formation of water trees and movement of water from hydrated dentine, through the hybrid layer and adhesive, to the adhesive–composite interface is especially marked with chemically cured composites. It is thought that this occurs because chemically cured composites polymerise more slowly than light-cured composites, permitting additional time for the water diffusion process to occur. This results in the formation of water blisters along the adhesive–composite interface, reducing bond strengths.

- Resin–dentine bonds formed by self-etch adhesives may degrade over time by the processes of resin elution, hydrolytic degradation, enzyme attack and thermal and functional stresses (Inoue et al., 2005). This degradation may be more apparent in self-etch adhesives that are strongly acidic than in those that are mildly acidic. Adhesives that are strongly acidic behave like phosphoric acid in etch-and-rinse adhesives – the smear layer is completely removed and a hybrid layer several microns thick is formed. All hydroxyapatite within the hybrid layer is removed. Self-etch adhesives, which are more mildly acidic, only form a submicron-thick hybrid layer and remnants of hydroxyapatite remain around the exposed collagen fibrils. It is suggested that there is chemical interaction between the functional monomers of mild self-etch adhesives and the hydroxyapatite remaining within the hybrid layer, in addition to the micromechanical retention resulting from the resin infiltrating the hybrid layer. The formation of calcium salts of the functional monomers may protect the bond from degradation over time. Adhesives based on 10-methacryloxy decyl dihydrogen phosphate (10-MDP) form stronger, more stable calcium salts within the hybrid layer than those based on the functional monomer 4-methacryloxyethyl trimellitic acid (4-META) or 2-methacryloxyethyl phenyl hydrogen phosphate (phenyl-P).

Influence of Filler Particles

There is a trend to add glass filler particles to dentine adhesive systems. The fillers may release fluoride, improve handling and coating of cavity walls and floors, and reinforce the hybrid layer, helping prevent bond failure through this region. Further research is required to substantiate these claims.

Glass-ionomer Dentine Adhesive Systems

Conventional and resin-modified glass–ionomer cements have been used as intermediary bonding agents for composite resin and dental amalgam restorations (see Chapter 5, page 79). They have the clinical advantages of readily bonding to tooth substance, releasing fluoride and being simple to use. The bond to dentine is by means of the formation of a narrow "hybrid" layer, giving micromechanical retention, and through chemical ionic bonding between the carboxylate groups of the glass-ionomer cement and calcium ions of the hydroxyapatite crystals in the partially demineralised dentine. As the glass-ionomer cement is a viscous material with glass filler particles, it creates a high-strength, thick layer that acts as a stress-breaker, helping to resist the stresses generated by the polymerisation contraction of a bonded composite restoration.

Durability of Bonds

Hydrophobic resin-based adhesives form a strong and durable adhesive bond to enamel that does not significantly deteriorate with time. This is not true for the bond to dentine – degradation of the adhesive bond to dentine occurs over time (Pashley, 2004). The bond is challenged at inception by polymerisation contraction, and then by cyclic mechanical fatigue loads during mastication, thermal cycling, chemical degradation and water diffusion into the hybrid layer. Bacterial enzymes are also thought to contribute to breakdown of collagen fibrils. Self-etch adhesives are increasingly hydrophilic and are subject to increased water uptake. Three-step etch-and-rinse adhesives have been shown to be the most resistant to long-term degradation (De Munck et al., 2005a).

Clinical Performance of Dental Adhesives

The most popular method of assessing the clinical performance of dental adhesives is by comparing the retention of composite restorations in non-carious cervical lesions. The advantages of this model are that no tooth preparation is required, so eliminating a variable that is difficult to control, and failure of the adhesive bond will be obvious, with loss of restoration retention. Average annual failure rates of various types of dental adhesive vary greatly by material: glass-ionomer cements have a narrow range of values (0–7.6%) and self-etch one-step adhesives a very wide range (0–48%). A narrow range indicates a reliable material, whereas a wide range indicates increased technique sensitivity. Glass–ionomer adhesives give the best clinical performance, with etch-and-rinse three-step and self-etch two-step adhesives being clinically reliable and having predictably good performance.

References

Buonocore MG, Matsui A, Gwinnett AJ. Penetration of resin dental materials into enamel surfaces with reference to bonding. Arch Oral Biol 1968;13(1):61–70.

De Munck J, Van Landuyt K, Peumans M, Poitevin A, Lambrechts P, Braem M, Van Meerbeek B. A critical review of the durability of adhesion to tooth tissue: methods and results. J Dent Res 2005a;84(2):118–132.

De Munck J, Vargas M, Iracki J, Van Landuyt K, Poitevin A, Lambrechts P, Van Meerbeek B. One-day bonding effectiveness of new self-etch adhesives to bur-cut enamel and dentin. Oper Dent 2005b;30(1):39–49.

Inoue S, Koshiro K, Yoshida Y, De Munck J, Nagakane K, Suzuki K, Sano H, Van Meerbeek B. Hydrolytic stability of self-etch adhesives bonded to dentin. J Dent Res 2005;84(12):1160–1164.

Marshall GW Jr, Marshall SJ, Kinney JH, Balooch M. The dentin substrate: structure and properties related to bonding. J Dent 1997;25(6):441–458.

Nakabayashi N, Kojima K, Masuhara E. The promotion of adhesion by the infiltration of monomers into tooth substrates. J Biomed Mater Res 1982;16(3):265–273.

Nakabayashi N, Takarada K. Effect of HEMA on bonding to dentin. Dent Mater 1992;8(2):125–130.

Pashley DH. Smear layer: overview of structure and function. Proc Fin Dentl Soc 1992;88(Suppl 1):215–224.

Pashley DH, Tay FR, Yiu C, Hashimoto M, Breschi L, Carvalho RM, Ito S. Collagen degradation by host-derived enzymes during aging. J Dent Res 2004;83(3):216–221.

Tay FR, Pashley DH. Have dentin adhesives become too hydrophilic? J Can Dent Assoc 2003;69(11):726–731.

Chapter 4
Glass-ionomer Cements

Aim

The aim of this chapter is to provide information on the different types of glass-ionomer cements available and the unique properties of this group of materials.

Outcome

Readers will better comprehend how the composition and setting reaction of glass-ionomer cement dictates its handling to optimise clinical performance, including fluoride release, bond strength and dimensional stability.

Introduction

Glass-ionomer cement was first made commercially available in 1976 as a self-adhesive, tooth-coloured filling material called ASPA. It derived its name as an acronym of the major constituents, aluminosilicate glass and polyacrylic acid. The early materials were slow-setting and difficult to handle, with relatively poor aesthetics. Subsequently, there have been major improvements in the properties of this important group of materials.

Indications
Modern glass-ionomer cement is a versatile, "smart" dental material, with the following applications:
- definitive restorative material in low load-bearing areas in adults
- definitive restorative material for deciduous teeth
- provisional restorative material in adults
- core build-up material prior to crown placement
- liners and base
- luting cement for crowns, posts and bridges
- fissure sealant
- bonding agent for composite resins and dental amalgam.

Advantages

Glass-ionomer cements are popular materials as they display the following clinical advantages:

- they are tooth-coloured
- they bond chemically to tooth substance and non-precious metals without the need for additional adhesives
- they release fluoride
- their coefficient of thermal expansion is equivalent to that of tooth structure
- they have good biocompatibility.

Disadvantages

The advantages of glass-ionomer cements are offset by the following disadvantages:

- low fracture toughness, limiting applications in high load-bearing areas
- some types cannot be finished and polished at the same visit they are placed
- some types are vulnerable to acid erosion
- some types exhibit low flexural strength and wear resistance.

Types of Glass-ionomer Cement

Three main types of glass-ionomer cement are commonly used. They have different compositions and properties. These types are:

- conventional glass-ionomer cement
- conventional, high-viscosity, reinforced glass-ionomer cements (Fig 4-1)
- resin-modified glass-ionomer cements (Figs 4-2 and 4-3).

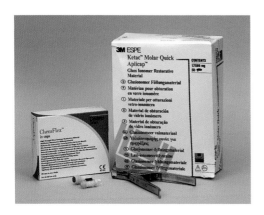

Fig 4-1 Examples of conventional high-viscosity or reinforced glass-ionomer cement, presented in capsules to be activated and mixed in an amalgamator.

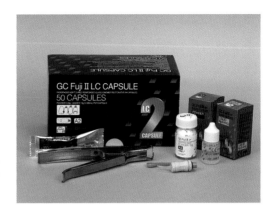

Fig 4-2 A resin-modified glass-ionomer cement, provided in both hand-mixed and capsulated versions.

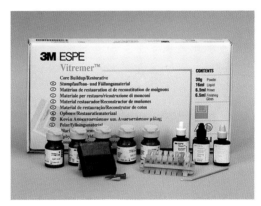

Fig 4-3 A resin-modified glass-ionomer cement, showing the range of shades available, powder:liquid formulation, conditioner and finishing gloss.

Conventional Glass-ionomer Cements

Glass Powders

Conventional glass-ionomer cements consist of an alkaline (basic) aluminosilicate glass with fluoride, which reacts with an acidic poly(alkenoic) acid to create a salt matrix and water. The glass filler particles are predominantly calcium aluminosilicate glasses, but certain manufacturers replace some of the calcium with strontium or lanthanum to increase cement radiopacity. An increase in radiopacity makes it easier for the clinician to identify the presence of recurrent caries under a restoration in a radiograph. Many different types of glasses are used, but the essential formulae are:

$$SiO_2–Al_2O_3–CaF_2 \text{ or } SiO_2–Al_2O_3–CaO$$

The glasses receive heat treatment during manufacture. This treatment alters surface reactivity of the powder, as does the particle size. A reduction in particle size increases reactivity, giving improved physical properties. Traditional glass-ionomer cements contained particles of up to 45 µm diameter. In modern materials this has been reduced to 1–15.5 µm.

Fluoride is present in the glass powder as calcium and sodium fluoride. Initially, it was added as a flux and to improve handling properties. The presence of the fluoride ion contributes to the formation of complex bodies with the metallic ions, released in to the liquid during the setting reaction. CaF^+ and AlF^{2+} are formed, which delay the bonding of the metallic cations with either polyacrylic acid – to form calcium and aluminium polyacrylate – or with the COO^- groups in the copolymer chains. This has the effect of slowing initial setting by gelation and thereby the working time is lengthened. Fluoride represents approximately 20% of the final glass powder. When the cement is mixed and set, the majority of the fluoride is released from the newly formed salt matrices.

Polyalkenoate Acid
The liquids are high molecular weight electrolytes based on homopolymers of acrylic acid or copolymers with itaconic or maleic acids. Copolymers were developed to improve the shelf life of the liquid, which had a tendency to become too viscous and inappropriate for use after about six months storage. The physical properties of a glass-ionomer cement can be improved by increasing the molecular weight or the concentration of the polyalkenoate acid.

Benefits attained are, however, limited by the fact that the cement becomes too viscous to be clinically useful above certain levels. Some manufacturers have mitigated the effects of this by freeze-drying the acid and adding it as a component in the powder, to be mixed with water alone or a mixture of water and tartaric acid.

Tartaric Acid
The addition of 5–10% of optically active L-tartaric acid improved the handling properties of the cement by delaying initial setting, similar to the action of fluoride, and then providing a rapid onset reaction. The clinical benefits of this are that it gives the clinician longer to manipulate the cement into the cavity and place a matrix if required, whilst shortening the length of time required for the material to set. In addition it increases the compressive strength of the cement (Nicholson, 1998).

Water

Water is an essential component of glass-ionomer cement. This distinguishes glass-ionomer cement from the majority of other tooth-coloured restorative materials, which are polymer based and hydrophobic. Between 11 and 24% of the set glass-ionomer cement is water, some "loosely" bound, some "tightly" bound. The loosely bound water is easily lost if the relative humidity surrounding a newly placed restoration falls below 70%. This is clinically critical, because if the cement is allowed to dehydrate, the loosely held water is lost very rapidly by evaporation, leading to excessive shrinkage. This shrinkage causes the cement to crack, compromising aesthetics and the physical properties of the cement. Cement dehydration is most likely to occur if the cement is isolated under a rubber dam, or is finished or polished with rotary instruments without the application of water coolant (see Chapter 7, pages 109-110). Slower setting aesthetic glass-ionomer cements are vulnerable to dehydration for up to six months after placement, while the faster-setting materials are less vulnerable after two weeks.

Glass-ionomer cement may also be damaged if exposed to excess water early after mixing and placement. Calcium and aluminium cations required for the setting reaction (see below) can be eluted in the presence of excess water, which interferes with the setting reaction, producing weak, unaesthetic cement with a chalky surface. Therefore, the surface of newly placed glass-ionomer cement must be protected from damage by saliva or premature mouth rinsing. Covering the setting cement with a matrix and isolating the tooth with cotton wool rolls, together with low-volume suction, most easily achieves this. Immediately the matrix is removed, a protective layer of low-viscosity methacrylate-based resin sealant or surface gloss should be applied to the surface of the cement and light-cured (Fig 4-4). Alternative materials for this use include petroleum jelly, copal or other proprietary varnishes, but they have a tendency to become porous and, as a consequence, relatively ineffective.

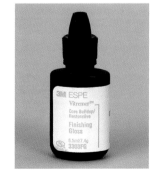

Fig 4-4 Example of a finishing gloss to be applied to the surface of a newly placed conventional glass-ionomer cement to prevent dehydration-induced structural damage.

Setting Reaction

The setting reaction of conventional glass–ionomer cement is shown in Fig 4-5. When the powder and liquid are mixed together the acid goes into solution. H^+ ions are released, which react with the outer layer of the fluoroaluminosilicate glass, releasing calcium, aluminium, sodium and

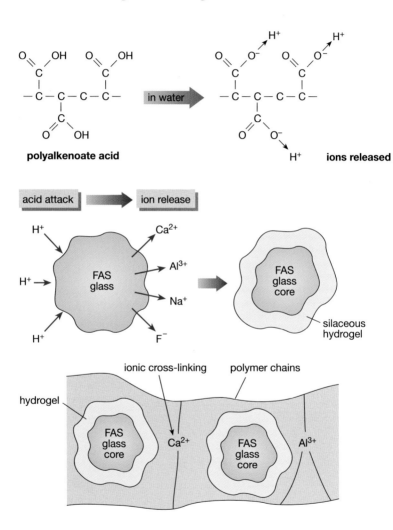

Fig 4-5 The setting reaction of conventional glass–ionomer cement by ionic cross-linking: FAS = fluoroaluminosilicate glass.

fluoride ions. This is called the "dissolution phase". The loss of the ions converts the outer layer of the glass particles into a siliceous gel. The calcium ions are released most rapidly and form calcium polyacrylate salt, initiating the setting reaction, known as the "gelation phase". At this stage the cement is very vulnerable to loss of calcium and aluminium ions if exposed to excess water, and it must therefore be kept isolated. It is also important that the powder and liquid are rapidly mixed and placed in the cavity prior to the commencement of the gelation phase. If the newly mixed cement has lost its surface gloss, the gelation phase has commenced and further manipulation by prolonged mixing or placement into a cavity will disrupt the delicate structure, leading to a compromised restoration with inferior physical properties.

The "hardening phase" follows the gelation phase. This process can take several days to complete. In this phase the aluminium complexes, including AlF^{2+}, form ionic cross-linkages with the acid, forming an aluminium polyacrylate salt matrix as the cement hardens. The precipitation of salts, in particular aluminium polyacrylate, continues for over 24 hours, and the cement becomes more transparent. It is after 24 hours has elapsed that the cement becomes significantly less soluble. At this time even the slowest-setting cements can be trimmed and polished, with the application of water coolant to avoid excessive frictional heat and dehydration. Faster-setting cements can be finished and polished 10 minutes after mixing, assuming application of water coolant in the process. It has been shown that the setting reaction continues at an almost imperceptible rate for up to 12 months after placement (Fricker et al., 1991).

The final microstructure of the set glass-ionomer cement is partially degraded glass particles surrounded by a layer of siliceous gel held in matrices of calcium and aluminium polyalkenoate (Fig 4-6).

Conventional Reinforced Glass-ionomer Cements

Many attempts have been made to overcome the disadvantages of glass-ionomer cements while retaining their advantages. Around 1985, "cermets" became available. These materials were glass-ionomer cements sintered with silver. Commercial examples were Ketac-Silver (ESPE) and Miracle Mix (GC International). Unfortunately, these materials, apart from having a metallic appearance, had low fracture toughness, which made them unsuitable for use in direct load-bearing areas.

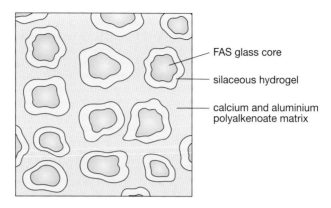

FAS glass core

silaceous hydrogel

calcium and aluminium polyalkenoate matrix

Fig 4-6 The structure of set conventional glass-ionomer cement: FAS = fluoroaluminosilicate glass.

In the late 1990s, significant modifications were made to the composition of conventional glass-ionomer cements, resulting in reinforced materials with improved compressive and flexural strength, hardness, wear resistance and solubility. This was achieved by increasing the powder:liquid ratio and by optimising the polyacid concentration and molecular weight. Polyacrylic acid was added to the powder and the glass particle size reduced to around 3 μm. The clinical advantages of these materials are that they can be used in load-bearing areas, and given their high viscosity they can be "packed" or condensed into cavities, facilitating clinical handling (Fig 4-7). They have increased radiopacity, compared with non-reinforced glass-ionomer cements. This is helpful in diagnosing secondary caries in dental radiographs. Commercial examples of these materials include Ketac Molar (ESPE), Fuji IX (GC International) and ChemFlex (Dentsply). They are clinically indicated as a

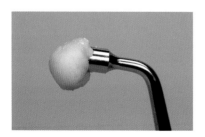

Fig 4-7 Mixed conventional reinforced glass–ionomer cement, showing how the material has a high viscosity and so can be formed into a ball and packed into a cavity using an amalgam packer.

lining material, for definitive restorations in deciduous teeth and in low stress-bearing areas in permanent teeth, as a long-term "temporary" restorative material, and as a core build-up material, in particular when the core acts as a transitional restoration. The clinical use of conventional reinforced glass-ionomer cement is illustrated in Figs 4-8 to 4-13.

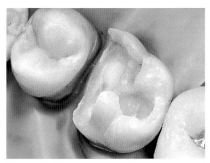

Fig 4-8 Cavity prepared on the mesial and occlusal surfaces of an upper left first molar. It is to be provisionally restored with a conventional reinforced glass-ionomer cement.

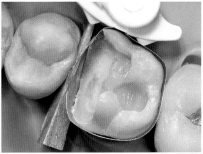

Fig 4-9 Cavity with metal matrix band held in place by a wooden wedge placed interproximally. The inner surface of the matrix band has a very thin layer of petroleum jelly applied, to prevent inadvertent bonding of the glass-ionomer cement to the matrix band.

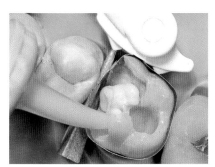

Fig 4-10 Conventional reinforced glass-ionomer cement, which has been mechanically mixed within a capsule, is syringed into the cavity.

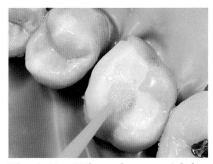

Fig 4-11 When the material has undergone an initial set, immediate application of finishing gloss to the surface of the conventional reinforced glass-ionomer cement helps prevent dehydration damage.

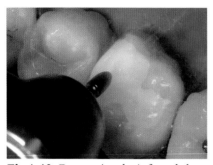 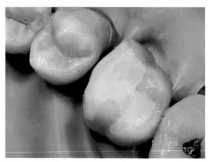

Fig 4-12 Conventional reinforced glass-ionomer cement being shaped with ultrafine finishing diamonds. Water coolant is applied to prevent dehydration of the surface of the material by heat generated by contact of the rotating bur with the restoration.

Fig 4-13 Finished conventional reinforced glass-ionomer cement in upper left first molar tooth.

Resin-modified Glass-ionomer Cements

Resin-modified glass-ionomer cements were first introduced in the late 1980s. Again, the aim was to retain the clinical advantages of conventional glass-ionomer cements, while improving compressive and flexural strength, fracture toughness and clinical handling. Further specific aims were to give the materials some degree of command-set through photopolymerisation, and the ability to be shaped and polished at the same visit they are placed. These aims were achieved by the addition of 2-hydroxyethyl methacrylate (HEMA) to the material. This could either be as a simple mixture, giving a photopolymerised HEMA matrix intermingled with the calcium and aluminium polyacrylate salt matrix of the acid–base setting reaction, or with photopolymerisable groups grafted onto polyacid chains.

The polymerisation of HEMA to poly-HEMA is usually photoinitiated by camphorquinone. Some materials, however, contain reduction/oxidation catalyst systems, such as micro-encapsulated potassium persulphate and ascorbic acid, which permit the polymerisation to occur in the absence of light (Vitremer, 3M ESPE). The clinical advantage of this is that the material can be placed in bulk; for example, as a core build-up material. The progression of the chemically cured acid–base setting reaction, together with the polymerisation reaction ensures that the material sets completely, even in areas where the curing light cannot adequately penetrate. The set cement contains approximately 5–7% HEMA.

Initially, there was confusion regarding the nomenclature of this group of materials of diverse composition and properties. Today, it is generally recognised that the materials that set by an acid–base reaction in an aqueous environment together with a polymerisation reaction are resin-modified glass-ionomer cements. This definition distinguishes resin-modified glass-ionomer cements from compomers – which are single-paste systems that include the major constituents of composite resins and glass-ionomer cements but do not contain water and, as a result, have a very limited acid–base setting reaction, limiting the ability to release fluoride (McCabe, 1998).

Setting Reaction

The setting reaction of resin-modified glass-ionomer cement is illustrated in Fig 4-14. These cements undergo at least two setting reactions, and in the case of some commercially available materials, three reactions. The first setting reaction is the conversion of HEMA to poly-HEMA when the cement is exposed to visible light. The exposure results in camphorquinone photoinitiators forming a methacrylate matrix around the aluminosilicate glass particles. This reaction causes the immediate hardening of the cement, resulting in favourable physical properties and permitting early finishing and polishing (with the application of water coolant). These procedures can be carried out within 10 minutes of mixing. The second setting reaction is the acid–base reaction between the aluminosilicate glass and polyalkenoic acid components of the material, as described for conventional glass-ionomer cements.

Newly placed resin-modified glass-ionomer cement requires protection from dehydration and cation elution by early exposure to water or saliva, as is required by conventional glass-ionomer cements. The presence of the HEMA matrix toughens the structure, but a protective layer of low-viscosity methacrylate-based resin sealant or surface gloss should still be applied to the surface of the newly placed cement and light-cured. The setting reaction of resin-modified glass-ionomer cement is still not fully understood, but there appears to be some degree of cross-linking between the poly-HEMA and polyalkenoate matrices that surround the unreacted glass particle cores in the set cement. In some materials, any HEMA which does not receive sufficient light to photopolymerise in the depths of the cavity can undergo a third, "dark-cure", setting reaction.

The hypothetical structure of set resin-modified glass-ionomer cement is illustrated in Fig 4-15.

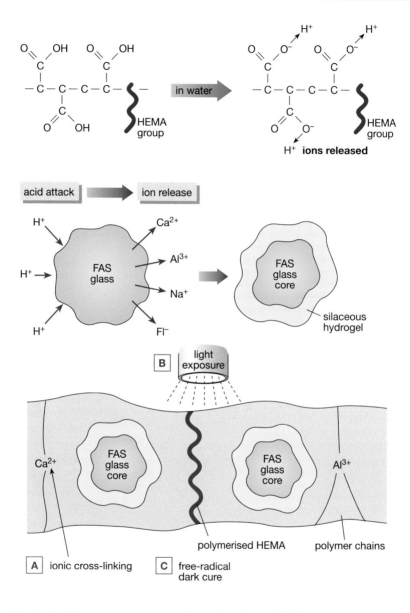

Fig 4-14 The three setting reactions of resin-modified glass-ionomer cement: A = ionic cross-linking, B = photopolymerisation when exposed to light, C = free-radical cure, which proceeds in the dark, FAS = fluoroaluminosilicate glass, HEMA = hydroxyethyl methacrylate.

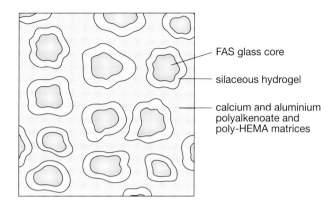

Fig 4-15 The set structure of resin-modified glass-ionomer cement: FAS = fluoroaluminosilicate glass, HEMA = hydroxyethyl methacrylate.

Disadvantages

The disadvantages of resin-modified glass-ionomer cements include the following:

- Resin-modified glass-ionomer cements contain HEMA, which increases the risk of a patient or member of the dental team having an allergic reaction.
- HEMA is strongly hydrophilic and absorbs water, leading to expansion. Under certain clinical circumstances, for example when used as the luting cement for an all-ceramic crown, this can lead to cracking of the restoration.
- Trimming and polishing must be carried out under water coolant to avoid dehydration and excessive shrinkage of the cement.
- Older formulations of resin-modified glass-ionomer cement discolour, in particular in patients with poor oral hygiene.

Bond Strength and Adhesion

Glass-ionomer cements demonstrate the significant advantage of being able to bond to enamel and dentine, stainless steel and non-precious metals with an oxide layer, without the need for the application of a separate bonding agent. When the newly mixed cement is applied to dentine, a narrow ion-exchange layer, 1–2 μm thick, is formed, which represents a chemical bond. This layer has been called an "intermediate" layer. Under transmission electron microscopy, a gradual transition can be seen as the collagen fibrils of dentine merge into the intermediate layer, and then into the bulk of the glass–ionomer cement.

It is suggested that the polyalkenoic acid diffuses into the tooth structure and displaces phosphate ions. To maintain electrolytic balance, each phosphate ion takes with it a calcium ion, which diffuses into the cement adjacent to the tooth, leading to the development of the ion-rich layer. The bond strength of glass–ionomer cement to dentine or enamel has never been measured, because when a displacing force is applied the cement always fails cohesively (just within the cement), leaving the intermediate layer on the surface of the tooth. Thus, what is measured, and sometimes erroneously reported as the adhesive strength of glass–ionomer cement to tooth, is actually the cohesive strength of the cement.

The bond can, however, be compromised if the surface is heavily contaminated with blood or saliva. Under these circumstances the surface should be cleaned using flours of pumice mixed to a slurry with water and applied with a bristle brush or prophylaxis cup. Application of 10% polyacrylic acid for 10 s followed by washing and gentle drying will clear surface debris with minimal demineralisation, exposing collagen fibrils and providing micromechanical retention to complement the chemical adhesion. Reports of the effects of the application of polyacrylic acid are equivocal, with some indicating increases in bond strength, and others indicating no increase. Its use is not essential in clinical practice, as adhesive failures of glass–ionomer cement restorations are uncommon.

Dynamic interactions occur between glass–ionomer cement and deep, hydrated dentine. Water diffuses from the wet dentine across the adhesive interface and just into the intermediate layer (Watson et al., 1998). Air voids within glass–ionomer cement, immediately adjacent to dentine, contain water permeated from the dentine. This water causes a continuation of the glass–ionomer reaction, forming hollow spherical bodies which are silicon-rich.

Clinical Performance

When considering the performance of restorations in non-carious cervical cavities, the use of glass–ionomer cements results in the highest retention rates and the most durable restorations (Peumans et al., 2005).

Dimensional Stability

Conventional glass-ionomer cements undergo 2–3% contraction on setting, over a short time interval. In clinical situations where the cement is bonded in thin layers, and therefore not free to undergo plastic deformation, this can lead to spontaneous cohesive fracture of the cement (Mitchell et al., 1995). A clinical example of this is when a glass-ionomer luting cement is used to bond a post within a post channel, or to cement a full-coverage crown. Resin-modified glass-ionomer cements are subjected to an additional small contraction when the HEMA resin component is photopolymerised. Resin-modified glass-ionomer cements, however, exhibit significantly higher fracture toughness compared with conventional glass-ionomer cements and as a result they are better able to resist the stress generated by contraction (Mitchell et al., 1999).

Subsequently, water uptake in environments of adequate relative humidity compensates for this shrinkage. Early formulations of resin-modified glass-ionomer lining and luting cements contained relatively high concentrations of HEMA, which is hydrophilic. These materials showed excessive water absorption, and expansion in excess of the setting contraction (Watts et al., 2000). This raised concerns regarding the suitability of resin-modified glass-ionomer cements as a core build-up material. If the core were placed and prepared for a crown in one visit, and an impression recorded, there would be a risk that subsequent dimensional changes of the core would interfere with the seating of the crown. This does not appear to be a problem with current glass-ionomer cement formulations.

Concerns have also been raised regarding the fracture of all-ceramic crowns when cemented with resin-modified glass-ionomer luting cement. Again, earlier luting cement formulations appeared more susceptible to hydrophilic expansion, and when combined with a non-reinforced ceramic restoration the potential for crown fracture existed. For that reason, resin-modified glass-ionomer luting cements are not generally recommended for the cementation of all-ceramic crowns.

Methods of Mixing

Glass-ionomer cements are available for hand or mechanical mixing. Hand-mixed versions require the powder and liquid to be measured out, typically using a spoon for the powder and a dropper to dispense the liquid. They are then mixed together on a paper pad using a plastic spatula. Hand-mixed versions are less expensive to use than equivalent mechanically mixed cements, which require additional mixing and extrusion devices. Hand-mixed cements have, however, the potential for errors in the powder:liquid ratio. Such errors compromise the mechanical properties of the cement.

Mechanically mixed cements have the powder and liquid accurately preproportioned by the manufacturer and supplied in a capsule. Capsules are activated by pressure, releasing the liquid into contact with the powder. The capsule is then placed in an amalgamator to be mixed by a linear oscillating action, or in a rotary device (RotoMix, 3M ESPE) to be mixed at a centrifugal frequency of 2950 rpm for 3 s. The RotoMix device rotates the capsule around an 80 mm diameter orbit, while the capsule holder rotates around its own axis. Quantification of the resultant porosity has shown that the size, number and volume of bubbles in specimens of some luting cements produced from encapsulated materials are significantly greater than in equivalent hand-mixed materials. There is, however, no significant difference in porosity for high-viscosity, restorative-grade glass–ionomer cements. Porosity or air bubbles within a cement will weaken it and produce areas of high stress, where cracks will initiate and propagate, compromising the clinical performance.

Fluoride Release

It is generally accepted that glass–ionomer cements help prevent secondary caries. A systematic review has shown, however, that there is no conclusive evidence for or against inhibition of secondary caries by glass–ionomer cement restorations. Some studies indicated that the use of glass–ionomer cement did help prevent the development of secondary caries around restoration margins and some did not (Randall and Wilson, 1999). Fluoride released from conventional and resin-modified glass–ionomer cements is similar, although significant variations are observed between different products. Fluoride release by compomers is significantly lower than from glass–ionomer cements, but is significantly higher than from fluoride-containing composite resins.

A review of laboratory-based studies, however, provided stronger evidence in support of reduction in secondary caries by glass–ionomer cement (Forsten, 1998). It was concluded that conventional and resin-modified glass–ionomer cements gave an initial burst of fluoride release, which then gradually reduced to a constant level. It was hypothesised that the anticariogenic effect of fluoride released from glass–ionomer cement occurred due to remineralisation of dentine and enamel directly surrounding the restoration, and because of a reduction in the type and number of bacteria inadvertently left on the cavity floor or in plaque subsequently deposited on the restoration surface.

The review also concluded that glass-ionomer cement restorations could be "recharged" with fluoride when applied in high concentration to the surface of the cement. This fluoride would be available for subsequent release. In addition, when the fluoride ions are released, there is a return of calcium and phosphate ions into the glass-ionomer to maintain electrolytic balance, leading to maturation and hardening of the cement surface. Further clinical studies would be required to demonstrate if these laboratory findings apply to glass-ionomer cements in clinical service.

References

Forsten L. Fluoride release and uptake by glass-ionomers and related materials and its clinical effect. Biomaterials 1998;19(6):503–508.

Fricker J, Hirota K, Tamiya Y. The effects of temperature on the setting of glass ionomer (polyalkenoate) cements. Aust Dent J 1991;36(3):240–242.

McCabe JF. Resin-modified glass-ionomers. Biomaterials 1998;19(6):521–527.

Mitchell CA, Douglas WH, Cheng YS. Fracture toughness of conventional, resin-modified glass-ionomer and composite luting cements. Dent Mater 1999;15(1):7–13.

Mitchell CA, Orr JF, Kennedy JG. Factors influencing the failure of dental glass ionomer luting cement due to contraction. Biomaterials 1995;16(1):11–16.

Nicholson JW. Chemistry of glass-ionomer cements: a review. Biomaterials 1998;19(6):485–494.

Peumans M, Kanumilli P, De Munck J, Van Landuyt K, Lambrechts P, Van Meerbeek B. Clinical effectiveness of contemporary adhesives: a systematic review of current clinical trials. Dent Mater 2005;21(9):864–881.

Randall RC, Wilson NH. Glass-ionomer restoratives: a systematic review of a secondary caries treatment effect. J Dent Res 1999;78(2):628–637.

Watson TF, Pagliari D, Sidhu SK, Naasan MA. Confocal microscopic observation of structural changes in glass-ionomer cements and tooth interfaces. Biomaterials 1998;19(6):581–588.

Watts DC, Kisumbi BK, Toworfe GK. Dimensional changes of resin/ionomer restoratives in aqueous and neutral media. Dent Mater 2000;16(2):89–96.

Chapter 5
Dental Amalgam

Aim

Amalgam is one of the most established materials for the restoration of posterior teeth, but recently its use has been challenged because of health and environmental concerns. The aim of this chapter is to increase knowledge of dental amalgam, including its use with enamel and dentine adhesive systems in the bonded amalgam technique.

Outcome

Readers will gain insight into the indications, advantages and disadvantages of amalgam, including its safe use and disposal.

Introduction

In many countries, dental amalgam continues to be one of the most widely used dental materials for the restoration of posterior teeth. It has been successfully used for over 170 years, with favourable cost-effectiveness and clinical durability. Dental amalgam is, however, unaesthetic and lacks the ability to bond to remaining tooth tissues.

Indications

Amalgam is primarily indicated for the restoration of occlusal and occlusoproximal cavities in posterior teeth. It also continues to find application as a core build-up material prior to preparing a tooth for a crown. The use of dental amalgam is falling internationally, with the application of tooth-coloured alternatives increasing steadily.

Advantages
- cost-effective
- less technique-sensitive than composite resin
- high clinical survival rates (durability)
- fewer allergic or hypersensitivity reactions than composite resin
- strong evidence base.

Disadvantages

- unsightly restorations
- does not bond to tooth substance, requires mechanical retention and resistance features
- relatively low tensile strength, weak in thin (<2 mm) sections
- few, if any, applications in minimally interventive dentistry
- concerns regarding mercury as a potential toxin and environmental contaminant.

Composition

Dental amalgam is created when mercury is mixed, or triturated, with metal alloys. The composition of the metal alloys used has changed with time. Zinc-free and, in particular, high-copper alloys now predominate. The compositions of conventional (low-copper) and high-copper amalgam alloys are given in Table 5-1. In addition to the major elements, alloys may also contain small amounts of palladium, platinum, indium and gold.

Modern dental amalgam alloys may be classified as admixed high-copper alloys or single-composition high-copper alloys. As the alloy composition varies, so does the setting reaction. The metal alloy powder is triturated with liquid mercury in a sealed plastic capsule (Fig 5-1) using a mechanical triturator or amalgamator (Fig 5-2).

The mixing process produces a soft silver pellet of dental amalgam, which is condensed in increments into the cavity using a hand-held amalgam condenser. For condensation of the amalgam to be effective, amalgam

Table 5-1 **Composition of conventional (low-copper) and high-copper amalgam alloys**

Component	Conventional amalgam (% by weight)	High-copper amalgam (% by weight)
Silver	63–70	40–70
Tin	26–28	22–30
Copper	2–5	13–40
Zinc	0–2	0–2

condensers must be firmly applied to adapt the material and remove excess mercury. Given the need to firmly condense amalgam, matrices must be secure and well wedged if marginal excesses are to be avoided.

When triturated, mercury dissolves silver and tin from the metal alloy particles to form matrices of intermetallic compounds that bind the silver–tin particles (gamma phase) together into a solid set mass. The details of the setting reaction vary with the type of alloy used.

Amalgam Trituration
- Overtrituration produces a hot, sticky mix with decreased working and setting time and slightly increased setting contraction.
- Undertrituration produces a grainy, crumbly mix, which cannot be used.

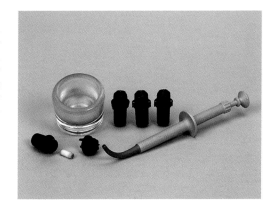

Fig 5-1 Example of amalgam capsules which contain preproportioned mercury liquid and amalgam alloy powder, together with a small plastic pestle that mixes the components together when the capsule is mechanically mixed in an amalgamator. Also shown are a dappen dish, used to hold the triturated amalgam, and a plastic amalgam carrier, used to syringe the mixed amalgam into a prepared cavity.

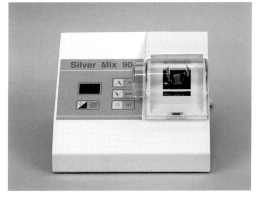

Fig 5-2 Example of a dental amalgamator, used to mechanically mix amalgam capsules containing preproportioned mercury liquid and amalgam alloy powder. Note the clear plastic lid, which should be closed during mixing to minimise any release of mercury vapour.

Conventional (Low-copper) Alloys

On trituration, a conventional (low-copper) alloy with a silver–tin alloy (gamma phase) releases tin and silver, which react with mercury to form silver–mercury (gamma 1) and tin–mercury (gamma 2) phases (Figs 5-3a and 5-3b).

$$\underset{\text{gamma}}{Ag_3Sn} \quad + \quad \underset{\text{mercury}}{Hg} \quad \longrightarrow \quad \underset{\text{gamma}}{Ag_3Sn} \quad + \quad \underset{\text{gamma 1}}{Ag_2Hg_3} \quad + \quad \underset{\text{gamma 2}}{Sn_8Hg}$$

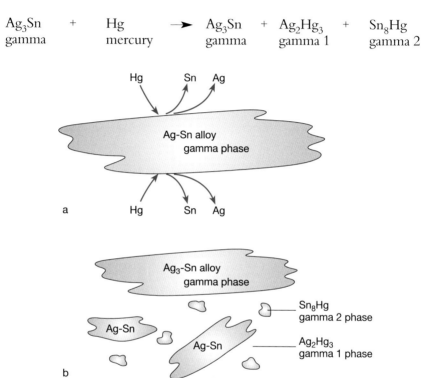

Fig 5-3 (a) The interaction between mercury and a conventional (low-copper) amalgam alloy. The outer aspects of the silver–tin alloy particles (gamma phase) dissolve in the mercury, releasing tin and silver. (b) The compounds formed by the release of silver and tin, primarily gamma 1 phase (Ag_2Hg_3) and gamma 2 phase (Sn_8Hg). The final structure of a set, low-copper amalgam consists of large amounts of unreacted gamma phase (Ag_3-Sn), together with smaller amounts of gamma 1 and gamma 2 phases.

Admixed High-copper Alloys

When triturated, tin moves to the surface of the silver–copper alloy particles and reacts with the higher copper content to create a new copper–tin (eta phase), which surrounds the unreacted cores of the silver–copper particles. These particles are bound together with silver–mercury (gamma 1) phase (Figs 5-4a and 5-4b). Thus, there is almost no gamma 2 phase in these amalgams, which is weak and susceptible to corrosion.

$$Ag_3Sn + Hg + AgCu \longrightarrow Ag_3Sn + Ag\text{–}Cu + Ag_2Hg_3 + Cu_6Sn_5$$
$$\text{gamma} \qquad\qquad\qquad\quad \text{gamma} \qquad\qquad \text{gamma 1} \quad\ \text{eta}$$

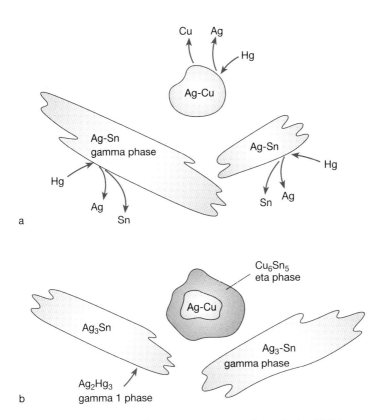

a

b

Fig 5-4 (a) The interaction between mercury and an admixed high-copper amalgam alloy. The mercury diffuses into the silver–copper particles, releasing silver and copper, while the silver–tin alloy particles (gamma phase) release silver and tin. (b) The mercury reacts with the silver–tin particles and forms gamma 1 (Ag_2Hg_3) and gamma 2 (Sn_8Hg) phases, as for a low-copper alloy, leaving some gamma phase (Ag_3Sn) unreacted. The newly formed gamma 2 phase reacts with the silver–copper particles to form Cu_6Sn_5 (eta phase). These reactions almost totally eliminate the gamma 2 phase, which is responsible for susceptibility to corrosion.

The actions of each amalgam alloy constituent are summarised in Table 5-2.

Table 5-2 **Actions of amalgam alloy constituents**

Constituent	Actions
Silver	Increases strength and expansion
Tin	Increases setting time, decreases strength and expansion
Copper	Increases strength, reduces corrosion, reduces creep, reduces amount of weak gamma 2 phase
Zinc	Used in manufacturing to reduce oxidation of other elements; may cause delayed expansion if contaminated with water
Indium	Decreases creep, increases strength, decreases surface tension and therefore reduces amount of mercury required
Palladium	Reduces corrosion

High-copper Alloys

High-copper alloys are now the most popular type of amalgam used, as they give high early compressive strength, low creep, good corrosion and marginal fracture resistance. These properties are obtained as the high copper content eliminates or greatly reduces formation of a tin–mercury phase (gamma 2), which weakens low-copper composition amalgam restorations and causes them to corrode.

Zinc-free Alloys

Previously, zinc was added to alloy compositions, in concentrations of 0–2% by weight, to aid casting of the alloy ingots (see below) by reducing oxidation of other elements. Most recent formulations contain less than 0.01% by weight of zinc. A higher level leaves an amalgam vulnerable to excessive delayed expansion following the release of hydrogen gas if the restoration is contaminated with moisture during condensation.

$$H_2O \quad + \quad Zn \quad \longrightarrow \quad ZnO \quad + \quad H_2$$
water   zinc   zinc oxide   hydrogen gas

74

Morphology of Alloys

Dental amalgam alloys may be cast into ingots and then reduced to filings by being cut on a lathe and reduced in size in a ball mill. These alloys are described as lathe-cut. The filings are typically 60–120 μm in length. An alternative method of production is to create spherical alloy particles by spraying the liquid alloy under high pressure in an inert gas through a fine crack in a crucible into a large chamber (Powers and Sakaguchi, 2006). Spherical particles vary in size from 2-43 μm. Some alloys contain a mixture of lathe-cut and spherical particles and are described as admixed.

Amalgams of lathe-cut alloys require firm pressure to condense. They benefit from the use of a small-diameter amalgam condenser. They have been shown to be better adapted to the cavity wall than spherical particle alloys. This has led to the suggestion that the relatively large interfacial gap typically associated with spherical alloys may lead to increased leakage and post-operative sensitivity compared with that observed with lathe-cut alloys.

Spherical alloy particles have a small surface area and require relatively little mercury to wet the surface. They are softer and require less pressure to condense than lathe-cut alloys, and benefit from the use of a broad-diameter amalgam packer. They harden rapidly and give a smooth polish. A disadvantage is that it is more difficult to achieve a tight interproximal contact in addition to the difficulties which may be associated with interfacial adaptation.

Admixed alloys are a popular choice, demonstrating properties between those of lathe-cut and spherical alloys. They give good interproximal contacts and polish, but their setting time may be too slow for experienced operators and they have low early strength.

Creep

Dental amalgam subjected to a continual compressive force undergoes permanent deformation, or creep. A low value of creep is desirable to minimise marginal breakdown in restorations. Creep values for different dental amalgams vary from 6.3% for low-copper lathe-cut alloys down to 0.05% for high-copper spherical alloys.

Dimensional Stability

An ideal restorative material is dimensionally stable, and does not contract or expand on setting. Amalgam undergoes an initial contraction, caused by the solution of mercury in the alloy particles, followed by a period of expansion. The net result is a small contraction. Amalgams that give the largest contraction on setting will result in larger interfacial gaps between the cavity wall and the restoration. This will predispose the interface to leakage, which if extensive or prolonged can lead to pulpal inflammation and post-operative sensitivity.

Contraction on setting can be offset by application of a cavity varnish or by the use of an amalgam bonding agent. In clinical service, corrosion products build up in the interface.

Amalgam Bonding

Dental amalgam does not bond to tooth substance. It is dependent on the creation of mechanical undercuts, slots, grooves or, to a lesser extent than practised previously, dentine pins to gain adequate retention and resistance form, to ensure that it is retained in the cavity. Creation of mechanical features such as undercuts and grooves may require undesirable sacrifice of sound tooth substance.

There are significant risks associated with the use of dentine pins. A small, but not insignificant, number of dentine pins accidentally perforate into the pulp or periodontal ligament, risking inflammation and necrosis. In addition, use of a pin twist drill without water coolant to prepare the pin channel has been shown to cause a rise in temperature that may endanger pulp vitality (Biagioni et al., 1996). Placement of dentine pins generates high levels of stress within the dentine, which can lead to crazing or dentine fracture. While pins help to retain an extensive amalgam, they tend to weaken the restored tooth unit.

Amalgam may be adhesively bonded to tooth substance using the bonded amalgam technique (Fig 5-5). Clinical studies have shown the technique to be successful, with the retention gained equalling that achieved with the dentinal pins. Amalgam bonding may reduce leakage and post–operative hypersensitivity and improve retention rates. Fracture resistance may, however, deteriorate with time.

The reduction in leakage achieved by amalgam bonding is of particular benefit in teeth that have undergone a direct or indirect pulp cap prior to placement of the amalgam. This benefit may be enhanced by the combined use of liners, bases and amalgam bonding, subject to sufficient dentine being available to achieve effective bonding.

The technique requires etching of the enamel and dentine to produce micromechanical bonding with enamel and a hybrid layer with dentine, as described in Chapter 3, pages 39–40. Many of the bonding agents indicated for this technique contain 4-methacryloxyethyl trimellitic acid (4-META) and a filler to produce a thick bonding layer of 20–50 μm (Anusavice, 2003).

The clinical technique is shown in Figs 5-6 to 5-14.

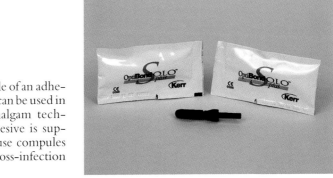

Fig 5-5 Example of an adhesive system that can be used in the bonded amalgam technique. The adhesive is supplied in single-use compules for improved cross-infection control.

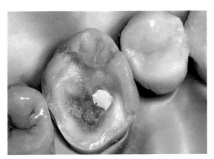

Fig 5-6 Cavity prepared on the distal, palatal and occlusal surfaces of an upper right first molar tooth. The cavity was very deep, and therefore a calcium hydroxide indirect pulp cap was placed prior to the photograph being taken.

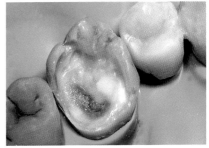

Fig 5-7 Calcium hydroxide lining covered with a thin layer of resin-modified glass-ionomer cement lining material. Care is taken to extend this lining only 1–2 mm beyond the calcium hydroxide lining, to ensure that a maximum surface area of dentine remains available for the bonded amalgam technique.

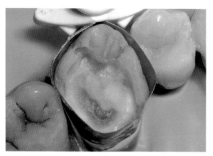

Fig 5-8 Cavity with metal matrix band held in place by a wooden wedge placed interproximally. The inner surface of the matrix band has a very thin layer of petroleum jelly applied, to prevent inadvertent bonding of the bonded amalgam to the matrix band.

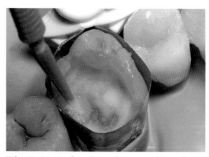

Fig 5-9 Orthophosphoric acid etchant being applied to the enamel and dentine of the prepared cavity. Care is taken to avoid etching the surface of the resin-modified glass-ionomer cement. The etchant is then washed away and lightly dried.

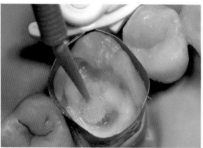

Fig 5-10 Enamel and dentine adhesive system being applied to the cavity with an applicator brush.

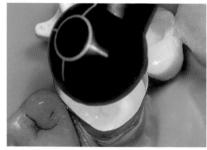

Fig 5-11 Photopolymerisation of the adhesive used in the bonded amalgam technique.

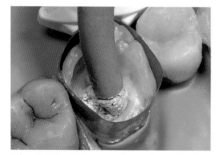

Fig 5-12 Triturated amalgam being placed in the prepared cavity.

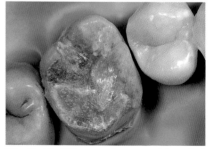

Fig 5-13 The newly carved bonded amalgam restoring an upper right first molar tooth.

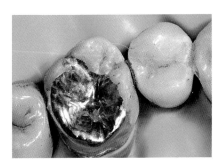

Fig 5-14 The surface of the newly placed bonded amalgam after burnishing.

Conventional and resin-modified glass-ionomer cements have been successfully used to bond amalgam to tooth substance (Chen et al., 2000). Freshly triturated amalgam is packed against a layer of uncured adhesive applied over the cement, causing physical intermingling of the amalgam with the bonding agent (Geiger et al., 2001). On setting, the amalgam is tethered in place by the bonding agent (Fig 5-15). It is advisable to avoid applying

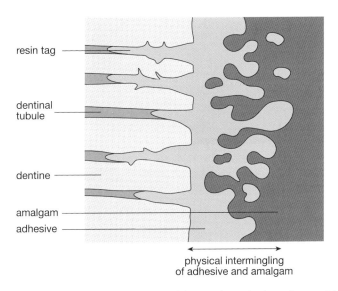

Fig 5-15 The physical intermingling of the newly packed amalgam with the surface of the adhesive, which in turn is micromechanically retained to the dentine by the hybrid layer and resin tags.

79

bonding agent to the surface of set amalgam if the technique is used as part of a repair procedure. The adhesive will interfere with the weak bond achieved when freshly triturated amalgam is condensed against set amalgam.

Amalgam bonding requires additional clinical time and the use of adhesive materials. It is justified in cavities that lack sufficient mechanical retention and resistance features, and which, without the use of a bonding agent, would require removal of additional tooth substance or placement of a dentine pin. It is also a useful adjunct in teeth to be crowned, where crown preparation will remove retentive features, leaving the amalgam core vulnerable to displacement.

Choosing an Amalgam

It is sensible to choose a high-copper, zinc-free dental amalgam. Operator preference normally influences the choice between lathe-cut, spherical or admixed alloys, but admixed alloys are by far the most popular. In addition, some alloys are available in regular- and slow-set formulations, with most practitioners opting for regular-set alloys, unless especially large restorations are to be placed. If there is a delay in packing an amalgam, excess mercury will not be brought to the surface to be removed during initial contouring. Excess mercury left in the amalgam leads to decreased compressive strength and increased creep. In addition, partially set amalgam increments will not bond to the previously packed amalgam, leading to increased amalgam porosity and poorer adaptation to the cavity walls. This may lead to fracture of the amalgam margins during carving and decreased amalgam strength, leaving the restoration susceptible to bulk fracture in clinical service.

Safe Use and Disposal

Concerns exist regarding the safe use of dental amalgam given its mercury content – elemental mercury being a toxic substance. Safety issues include mercury release in dental surgeries during the storage, trituration, placement, polishing and removal of dental amalgams (Eley, 1997). Small quantities of mercury are released when amalgam restorations are chewed or brushed, and the patient is exposed to mercury when amalgam fillings are placed and, in particular, removed. Much of the mercury entering the body is excreted, however small amounts remain in the kidneys, brain, lungs and gastrointestinal tract. It has been estimated that in the UK, one-sixth of mercury present in an adult is from amalgam restorations, with the rest coming from the environment, primarily through the consumption of fish

(fish are contaminated with mercury as a consequence of pollution of the world's oceans from industrial sources).

Given these concerns, much research has been carried out to determine the safety of dental amalgams and amalgam restorations. The World Health Organization, the FDI (World Dental Federation), the American Dental Association and the UK's Department of Health Committee on Toxicity of Chemicals in Food, Consumer Products and the Environment, among others, have found dental amalgam to be safe when used in accordance with manufacturers' directions. In contrast, in some countries, notably in Scandinavia, the use of dental amalgam has been substantially restricted, as part of wider measures to control the release of mercury into the environment. Contraindications to the use of dental amalgams have varied between countries and with time. They have typically included use in pregnancy, lactating mothers and young children. The issue of the safety of dental amalgam continues to be a matter of considerable debate around the world.

Contamination of the environment during disposal of waste amalgam into wastewater discharged from dental surgeries is of increasing concern. It has been calculated that an average dentist working full-time in general dental practice may be responsible for the discharge of 100–200 mg mercury per year. As a consequence, a number of countries, including the UK, have legislation making the installation of amalgam separators mandatory. These separators, which use sedimentation filters or centrifuges to remove amalgam from wastewater, have been shown to reduce mercury discharge by up to 90%.

Solid waste may also be contaminated with amalgam through the disposal of triturated amalgam capsules, used cotton wool rolls, dislodged amalgams and extracted teeth containing amalgam restorations. If this waste is incinerated, it gives rise to contamination of the atmosphere by bioavailable mercury vapour. Similarly, cremation of the deceased who had teeth restored with dental amalgams releases significant amounts of mercury vapour into the atmosphere. The environmental impact of this release continues to be actively researched. The impact of mercury contamination from dental sources should, however, be set in the context of global mercury release. Of this release, only 3–4% is estimated to be of dental origin, with the rest being caused by industrial pollution (Arenholt-Bindslev, 1998).

The dental team should take the following precautions when using dental amalgam to minimise the effects of exposure to mercury:

- Use encapsulated amalgams.
- Close cover of triturator when in use.
- Re-close capsules after use and store in a container designed for the purpose. These containers should be filled with water containing sodium thiosulphate.
- Avoid skin contact with amalgam.
- Use water spray and high-volume suction when removing old amalgams. Use of a rubber dam reduces mercury vapour exposure, in particular for the patient.
- Comply with legislation on use of amalgam separators to avoid contamination of wastewater.
- Avoid placement of amalgams during pregnancy and breastfeeding.
- Screen new members of the dental team for possible atypical reaction to mercury.
- Be familiar with the safe management of accidental spillage of mercury (Figs 5-16 and 5-17).

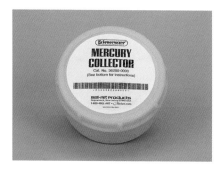

Fig 5-16 Example of a commercially available plastic container used to safely manage mercury spillage.

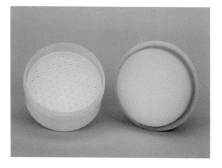

Fig 5-17 Contents of mercury spillage container. Attached to the undersurface of the lid is a foam pad. To safely collect spilled mercury, the lid is held and the foam pad pressed firmly onto the spill. This pressure forces the mercury into the pad. When the lid is screwed back onto the container, the foam pad is compressed against the container's free-standing perforated plate, releasing the mercury into the bottom of the container.

Adverse Reactions and Dental Amalgam

Annually, millions of dental amalgams are placed worldwide with very few adverse reactions reported. Hypersensitivity reactions reported include contact dermatitis and oral lichenoid lesions adjacent to amalgam restoration, often when restoring the buccal and lingual walls of posterior teeth. Reactions are thought mainly to be due to the toxic and allergenic potential of mercury within amalgam. Between 1905 and 1986, 41 cases of amalgam allergy were reported; 37 of these were a reaction to mercury, two to copper and two to silver (Veron et al., 1986).

Oral lichenoid reactions are thought to be due to amalgam constituents or corrosion products locally altering the antigenicity of basal keratinocytes of the oral mucosa. This triggers cell-mediated autoimmune damage. Diagnosis is usually made on the basis of presentation, histological appearance at biopsy, patch-testing for mercury sensitivity and proximity and distribution of lesions to amalgam restorations in the mouth. Patch-testing to mercury is difficult to interpret and may not be helpful in making a diagnosis. Lichenoid reactions can present as reticular, striated, atrophic, erosive or ulcerative lesions of the mucosa, with or without symptoms. The majority of lichenoid reactions are found on the buccal mucosa and lateral border of the tongue. Resolution of the oral lichenoid lesions on replacement of the dental amalgams with an alternative restorative material has been reported to be in the range of 37.5–100% of cases (Issa et al., 2004). Oral lichenoid lesions may also be caused by drugs, such as nonsteroidal anti-inflammatory drugs, or a reaction to other restorative materials, such as palladium-alloy-based crowns or composite resin.

References

Anusavice K. Phillip's Science of Dental Materials. St Louis, Missouri: Saunders, 2003.

Arenholt-Bindslev D. Environmental aspects of dental filling materials. Eur J Oral Sci 1998;106(2 Pt 2):713–720.

Biagioni PA, Hussey D, Mitchell CA, Russell DM, Lamey PJ. Thermographic assessment of dentine pin placement. J Dent 1996;24(6):443–447.

Chen RS, Liu CC, Cheng MR, Lin CP. Bonded amalgam restorations: using a glass-ionomer as an adhesive liner. Oper Dent 2000;25(5):411–417.

Eley BM. The future of dental amalgam: a review of the literature. Part 2: Mercury exposure in dental practice. Br Dent J 1997;182(8):293–297.

Geiger SB, Mazor Y, Klein E, Judes H. Characterization of dentin-bonding-amalgam interfaces. Oper Dent 2001;26(3):239–247.

Issa Y, Brunton PA, Glenny AM, Duxbury AJ. Healing of oral lichenoid lesions after replacing amalgam restorations: a systematic review. Oral Surg Oral Med Oral Pathol Oral Radiol Endod 2004;98(5):553–565.

Powers JM, Sakaguchi RL. Craig's Restorative Dental Materials. Chapter 11 Amalgam. In: Powers JM, Sakaguchi RL (eds). Craig's Restorative Dental Materials. St Louis, Missouri: Mosby Elsevier, 2006:235–267.

Veron C, Hildebrand HF, Martin P. Dental amalgams and allergy. J Biol Buccale 1986;14(2):83–100.

Chapter 6
Sealers, Lining and Base Materials

Aim

The recommended use of sealers, lining and base materials has radically changed in recent times. The aim of this chapter is to give increased appreciation of the relationship between leakage around restorative materials and the maintenance of pulp vitality.

Outcome

Readers will be aware of techniques to protect pulp vitality, including the placement of direct and indirect pulp caps. The flow diagrams will aid clinicians in their choice of a restorative regime.

Protecting the Vitality of the Dental Pulp

The primary aim of managing caries and other damage to teeth should be preservation of pulp vitality. This is often best achieved by minimising pulpal inflammation. Even relatively superficial damage can lead to pulpal inflammation and symptoms of hypersensitivity (Brannstrom and Lind, 1965), Fig 6-1a. Where this has occurred and restorative intervention is required, the second aim of management is to minimise further pulpal inflammation by atraumatic minimal intervention. The action of cutting a diseased or damaged tooth further traumatises the pulp by application of mechanical and thermal stresses (Fig 6-1b). Important factors include drill speed, type of bur, pressure applied, time in contact with dentine and the use of water coolant.

The third aim of management is to choose restorative materials and procedures that do not irritate the pulp through the release of chemicals capable of passing through the dentine and causing adverse reactions in the pulp (Fig 6-2a). The final aim of management is to avoid late-onset pulpal inflammation, caused by bacterial ingress between the restoration and the cavity wall, in the absence of marginal seal (Fig 6-2b).

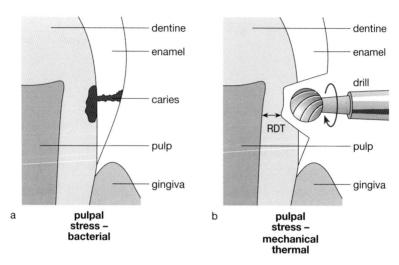

Fig 6-1 (a) The presence of a carious lesion may cause bacterial inflammation of the pulp. (b) Additional pulpal inflammation is caused by the action of cutting the tooth, which further traumatises the pulp by application of mechanical and thermal stresses: RDT = remaining dentine thickness.

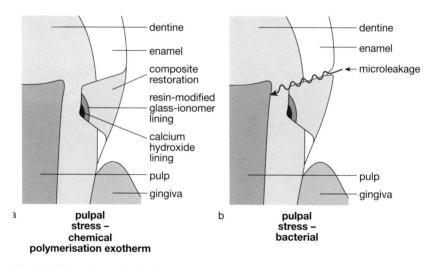

Fig 6-2 (a) Further pulpal inflammation may occur if lining and restorative materials are chosen that irritate the pulp by release of chemicals capable of passing through the dentine to the pulp. (b) Late-onset pulpal inflammation may take place if bacterial microleakage between the restoration and the cavity wall occurs.

Lining and base materials have important roles in preventing pulpal inflammation. The purposes of lining and base materials may include:

- Acting as a bacteriostatic agent against any bacteria present in carious dentine.
- Being biologically active and stimulating odontoblasts lining the pulp chamber to lay down tertiary dentine.
- Protecting the pulp by preventing diffusion of chemicals from the restorative material through dentine.
- Reducing leakage between the restoration and dentine.
- Isolating the pulp from intraoral thermal stimuli.
- Limiting fluid movement through dentine, which may give rise to symptoms of discomfort and pain.
- Providing rigid support for the overlying restorative material, in particular under loading.
- Blocking out undercuts if an indirect restorative technique is to be used.

Dentine is very effective at protecting the pulp from damage as it is a good insulator and reduces diffusion of chemicals from the cavity floor to the pulp (Stanley et al., 1975). An important factor in determining whether cavity preparation will cause pulpal change, by initiating secretion of a tertiary dentine matrix, is the remaining dentine thickness – the thickness of dentine between the floor of the cavity and the pulp. The preparation of shallow cavities, with 0.5–3.0 mm of remaining dentine thickness causes little irritation of the pulp, and therefore there is little stimulation of the odontoblasts to secrete reactionary dentine. The preparation of deep cavities, with 0.25–0.5 mm of remaining dentine thickness, causes a small reduction in numbers of odontoblasts following the injury, but maximally stimulates the surviving odontoblasts to lay down a thick layer of tertiary dentine. The preparation of very deep cavities, with 0.01–0.25 mm of remaining dentine thickness, causes greater trauma and a large reduction in odontoblast numbers. As a consequence, there are relatively few odontoblasts left to secrete tertiary dentine when it is most needed (Murray et al., 2002a).

Influence of Restorative Materials

Previously, it was thought that inflammation of the pulp was directly caused by toxins from restorative materials passing through the remaining dentine to the pulp. Now, it is thought that the effects of these chemicals are mild and short-lived, with pulpal irritation being caused by later-onset inflammation, induced by bacterial leakage (Watts and Paterson, 1987).

Under experimental conditions, when bacteria are excluded, most restorative materials cause little pulpal inflammation. In clinical service, however, it is almost impossible to prevent bacterial contamination of the tooth–restoration interface, with possible pulpal consequences. This leakage is often referred to in the literature as microleakage – the passage of bacteria, fluids, molecules or ions along the interface of a dental restoration and the wall of the cavity preparation. The ability to create a durable marginal seal and reduce microleakage varies according to the restorative material and the operative techniques employed.

Leakage

Restorative materials, including liners and bases, can protect the pulp by sealing the tooth from leakage or by their inherent bacteriostatic properties (or both).

- **Glass-ionomer cements** are good at limiting leakage as they bond chemically to both enamel and dentine. In addition, glass-ionomer cements are bacteriostatic, given their ability to release fluoride and other elements, notably zinc. There is a reduction in the number of cariogenic bacteria in the plaque adjacent to glass-ionomer restorations compared with restorations of composite resin or amalgam. The use of glass-ionomer cements, however, often in high caries-risk situations, does not preclude the possibility of bacterial leakage or secondary caries around restorations.

- **Composite resins** may intuitively be thought to be the best material to prevent leakage when bonded to enamel and dentine. However, even well-placed composite restorations will suffer at least some leakage over time, as resin bonds, in particular those to dentine, suffer some deterioration in clinical service. This can occur by water diffusion into the tooth–restoration interface, which causes breakdown of both the collagen and resin components of the hybrid layer (as discussed in Chapter 3, page 47). In addition, composite resins lack the ability to resist bacterial growth and the development of secondary caries. To limit such effects, it is essential to apply dental adhesives and composite resin strictly in accordance with manufacturers' directions, including the use of meticulous operative techniques.

- **Compomers** are not recommended by manufacturers for the restoration of cavities in teeth requiring a direct or indirect pulp cap. This is because some combinations of compomer and dentine adhesive do not give a reliable or durable marginal and interfacial seal as they demonstrate poor hybrid layer formation, short resin tags and interfacial and marginal porosities and gaps.

- **Amalgams**, although capable of being bonded to tooth substance, are typically placed without any provision to seal either margins or the tooth–restoration interfaces. Amalgams can, however, reduce leakage by the development of corrosion products at the cavity–amalgam interface, with the possibility of some antibacterial effects through the release of, among other elements, zinc, silver, copper and mercury.

Indirect and Direct Pulp Capping

If it is found during cavity preparation that caries is very deep, consideration should be given to indirect or direct pulp capping, to help preserve pulp vitality. The procedure is indicated when the tooth is asymptomatic and vital prior to the operative procedure and where there is no radiographic evidence of pulpal involvement. The tooth should be isolated by placing a rubber dam to minimise bacterial contamination of the cavity and, possibly, the pulp.

Caries is removed first from the enamel–dentine junction to determine whether the tooth is restorable. Under normal circumstances, if the caries extends more than 2 mm subgingivally the tooth will be unrestorable and will require extraction. If the tooth is judged restorable, possibly after crown lengthening, the next stage in cavity preparation is the removal of caries directly over the pulp. Soft, wet carious dentine is removed, but hard, possibly stained dentine may be left. This dentine is left to avoid pulpal exposure, which carries a high risk of bacterial contamination. If the pulp is contaminated with saliva or cavity debris, the prognosis for restoring pulp vitality is greatly reduced. A layer of hard-setting calcium hydroxide liner is then placed on the dentine. This layer of liner, which needs to be approximately 0.5 mm thick to be effective, has a number of actions, including antibacterial effects and the stimulation of reparative dentine. A clinical example of a calcium hydroxide lining in a deep cavity is shown in Fig 5-6. This is followed by the placement of a glass–ionomer base, covering just the calcium hydroxide and at least 0.5 mm of surrounding dentine. A well-adapted direct restorative material which offers marginal and interfacial seal is then placed (see Fig 5-7). This approach offers the best chance of the direct pulp cap being successful and pulp vitality being maintained.

The role of the glass–ionomer cement in this procedure is critical. Calcium hydroxide cement is weak and dissolves easily. It requires protection from mechanical forces, notably during restoration placement, and from dissolution over time, which leads to bacterial contamination and an increased risk of loss of pulp vitality. The glass-ionomer cement base is bacteriostatic and its ability to adhere to subjacent dentine limits subsequent leakage.

Is a Lining Necessary?

The material that best protects the pulp and maintains its vitality is dentine. Dentine insulates the pulp from temperature fluctuations and can prevent acids and other potentially toxic substances reaching the pulp. The thicker the dentine remaining between the cavity floor and the pulp, the better this protection will be. Sound dentine should never be removed to accommodate a liner or base.

Various materials can be placed on cavity floors and sometimes walls, prior to placement of a direct or indirect restoration. These are classified in order of increasing layer thickness:
- **Sealer:** such as varnishes or, more commonly, resin-based dentine.
- **Liner:** usually a resin or cement coating, around 0.5 mm thick, for example hard-setting calcium hydroxide or low-viscosity resin-modified glass-ionomer cement lining materials.
- **Base:** usually placed in layers greater than 0.5 mm thick, used for bulk build-up and blocking out undercuts in preparation for indirect restorations.

Sealers

Of the various forms of sealer available for direct application to prepared tooth surfaces, most interest in recent times has focused on resin-based sealers, used in the so-called "total-etch technique". This technique – which is now widely used in cavities of minimum and moderate depth to be restored with, in particular, a composite resin – involves acid etching of both enamel and dentine and the application of a resin-based adhesive. This technique, now increasingly and more helpfully referred to as the etch-and-rinse technique, has also been advocated as the sole form of pulp protection in deep cavities, but the evidence for the long-term effectiveness of this approach remains relatively limited. The term "wet bonding" is often linked to descriptions of etch-and-rinse techniques. Wet bonding, now more correctly referred to as "moist bonding", involves leaving the dentine slightly moist and glistening rather than excessively dehydrated and chalky in appearance. Moist bonding facilitates hybrid layer formation, while excessive drying may cause pulpal damage and compromise hybrid layer formation through collapse of the acid-etched exposed collagen network.

Liners

Of the various liners used in everyday clinical practice, hard-setting calcium hydroxide cements enjoy the greatest popularity. Calcium hydroxide is a very useful lining material because of its ability to stimulate deposition of reparative dentine and its biocompatibility. An example of a calcium hydroxide-based lining material is shown in Fig 6-3. Its success has been attributed to its antibacterial action and high pH, which reduces the causes of pulpal inflammation. In addition, calcium hydroxide may lead to growth factor release from dentine, stimulating new dentine formation and promoting pulpal healing (Murray et al., 2002b). The advantages of calcium hydroxide as a lining material are that it is:

- biologically active, stimulating new dentine formation
- bacteriostatic against bacteria present in carious dentine
- able to protect the pulp by preventing diffusion of noxious substances.

Unfortunately, calcium hydroxide cements have poor physical properties and are soluble, leading to loss of material under leaking restorations. This will leave the pulp vulnerably exposed to bacterial contamination. Calcium hydroxide linings must therefore be protected by a layer of glass-ionomer lining material.

The disadvantages of calcium hydroxide cements as a lining material include:

- Poor physical properties; they are therefore vulncrable to displacement at the time of restoration placement.

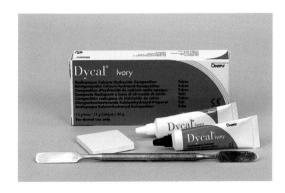

Fig 6-3 Example of a calcium hydroxide-based lining material.

- They are soluble in an aqueous environment.
- Poor thermal insulation of pulp from intraoral hot and cold stimuli.
- They do not bond to dentine, and as a consequence provide no barrier to leakage.
- They need to be protected by an overlying base, ideally one which bonds to dentine to provide protection.
- They do not provide support for the overlying restorative material.
- They cannot be used to block out undercuts in the provision of an indirect restoration.

Bases

Conventional and resin-modified glass-ionomer cements are excellent materials for the provision of a base. The advantages of these materials for this application include:
- They are bacteriostatic, limiting bacteria growth in any residual carious dentine.
- They provide thermal insulation of the pulp from intraoral hot and cold stimuli.
- They protect the pulp from the adverse effects of leachants from overlying restorative materials.
- They reduce leakage between the restorative filling material and dentine.
- They provide rigid support for the overlying restorative material.
- They are an excellent material for blocking out undercuts in the provision of indirect restorations.
- Composite resin bonds to the micromechanically rough surfaces of glass-ionomer cements.
- They can be used to help bond amalgam restorations in extensive preparations.

The disadvantages of glass-ionomer cements as lining materials include:
- They are not biologically active and do not stimulate odontoblasts lining the pulp chamber to lay down reparative dentine.
- They require space to be placed in a minimum effective thickness, around 0.5 mm.

An example of a resin-modified glass-ionomer cement base is shown in Fig 6-4.

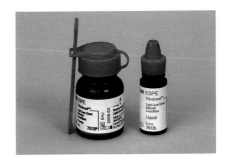

Fig 6-4 Example of a resin-modified glass-ionomer cement lining material.

How Should the Pulp be Protected?

Flow diagrams to aid the clinician to decide how best to protect the pulp are set out in Figs 6-5 to 6-7. These diagrams should be viewed as the best available,

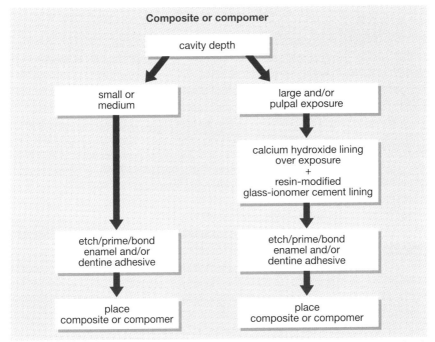

Fig 6-5 Flow diagram aiding choice of lining material dependent on cavity depth and whether pulpal exposure is present, when the cavity is to be restored with resin composite or compomer.

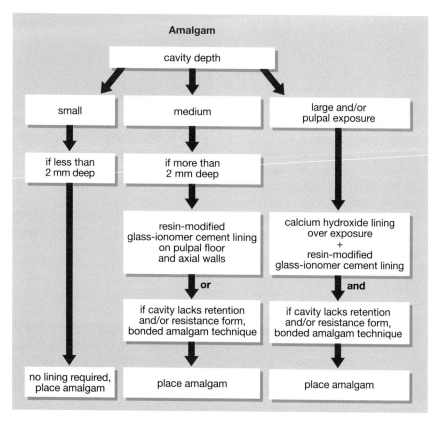

Fig 6-6 Flow diagram aiding choice of lining material dependent on cavity depth and whether pulpal exposure is present, when the cavity is to be restored with amalgam.

evidence-based guidance to pulp protection. Final decisions on pulp protection are influenced by circumstances specific to each case, such as whether the pulp has been exposed and which restorative material is to be used.

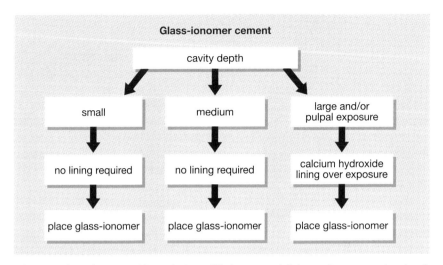

Fig 6-7 Flow diagram aiding choice of lining material dependent on cavity depth and whether pulpal exposure is present, when the cavity is to be restored with glass-ionomer cement.

References

Brannstrom M, Lind PO. Pulpal response to early dental caries. J Dent Res 1965;44(5):1045–1050.

Murray PE, About I, Lumley PJ, Franquin JC, Remusat M, Smith AJ. Cavity remaining dentin thickness and pulpal activity. Am J Dent 2002a;15(1):41–46.

Murray PE, Windsor LJ, Smyth TW, Hafez AA, Cox CF. Analysis of pulpal reactions to restorative procedures, materials, pulp capping, and future therapies. Crit Rev Oral Biol Med 2002b;13(6):509–520.

Stanley HR, Conti AJ, Graham C. Conservation of human research teeth by controlling cavity depth. Oral Surg Oral Med Oral Pathol 1975;39(1):151–156.

Watts A, Paterson RC. Bacterial contamination as a factor influencing the toxicity of materials to the exposed dental pulp. Oral Surg Oral Med Oral Pathol 1987;64(4):466–474.

Chapter 7
Finishing and Polishing Restorations

Aim

The aim of this chapter is to describe the armamentarium that can be used to finish and polish different types of restorative material.

Outcome

Readers will gain increased understanding of the best methods of finishing and polishing restorations, as determined by material type, filler particle size and restoration location.

Introduction

Finishing a restoration involves contouring to create optimal marginal finish, without overhangs or excess material extending beyond the cavity margin, and establishing an occlusal anatomy in harmony with the rest of the dentition. Polishing a restoration involves smoothing the surface with a series of abrasives to create the lowest surface roughness and a high surface lustre or polish.

The advantages of finishing and polishing include:
- minimising plaque accumulation at margins and on surfaces of restorations
- minimising the risk of surface staining
- minimising surface degradation and wear in clinical service
- maximising the aesthetics of the restoration by creating a high lustre or polish
- enhanced patient and dentist satisfaction
- reduced likelihood that a dentist will decide to replace the restoration unnecessarily (Oleinisky et al., 1996).

There are, however, some potential disadvantages of excessive finishing and polishing; a notable problem is increased heat generation, which may adversely affect the pulp.

Dental Amalgams

At placement, contouring of the amalgam is carried out using various instruments, according to the clinician's preference and the specific circumstances. Carving should always be across margins on to adjacent tooth tissue to optimise marginal adaptation. The surface of the carved amalgam should be lightly compacted and smoothed with a burnisher hand instrument. This technique, sometimes referred to as resurfacing, aims to homogenise the amalgam forming the surface of the restoration and to readapt the material to cavity margins – in particular, where it may have been carved away (see Fig 5-14).

The surface of the amalgam may be given a uniform lustre with a damp cotton wool pellet held in tweezers. This procedure aids refinements at a subsequent visit and improves marginal integrity. Excessive manipulation of the surface of a newly placed amalgam should be avoided to prevent gouging or damage to the structure.

At the next appointment, the surface of the amalgam can be refined, if required, using steel finishing burs, with water coolant to avoid overheating and to reduce the amount of mercury vapour released. Steel finishing burs are available in a range of sizes and shapes to aid access to all aspects of the restoration (Fig 7-1).

An exception to the normal protocol is high-copper amalgams with high early strength (see Chapter 5, page 74). Restorations of these amalgams may

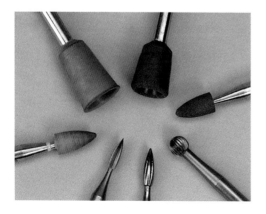

Fig 7-1 Examples of burs used to polish dental amalgam. Steel finishing burs are shown in the lower part of the picture, and "greenies'" and "brownies" – abrasive finishing points – in the upper part.

be polished 8–10 minutes after the start of trituration, to avoid the need for the patient to attend for a second appointment.

Polishing is a procedure that makes amalgam restorations look their best, but it makes little difference to clinical performance. Polishing can be carried out in a number of different ways. The traditional method entails polishing with flours of pumice, mixed with water, followed by zinc oxide powder in an alcohol slurry, applied using a prophylaxis cup in a low-speed handpiece. This is a low-cost option for polishing, but it has the disadvantage of splatter from the rotating cup, which can be very messy and unpleasant for the patient. These procedures produce a mirror-like surface finish on an amalgam.

Amalgam restorations may also be polished using rubber cups impregnated with abrasive particles (Fig 7-1) or aluminium oxide discs (see Fig 7-2). These devices should be used with water coolant to avoid excessive heat generation in the restored tooth.

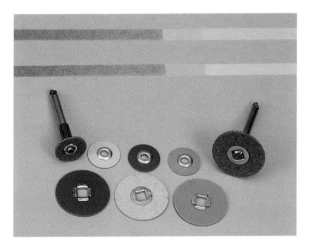

Fig 7-2 Examples of aluminium oxide abrasive discs and strips. Note the clear section in the centre of the strip, which contains no abrasive particles. This is the thinnest area, to aid movement of the strip through a tight dental contact point. The darker area to the left of the strip is more abrasive for shaping, and the lighter area to the right less abrasive for polishing. Smaller-diameter abrasive discs are useful in areas of limited access, such as around cervical cavities and palatally. Larger-diameter discs are useful for larger, flatter areas, such as when polishing extensive restorations involving the labial and incisal edge surfaces of anterior teeth.

Old, corroded amalgams with ditched margins that are restoring teeth free from caries may often be refurbished by recontouring with steel burs and polishing. This may restore a satisfactory surface finish and marginal adaptation, extending the life expectancy of the restoration. This is preferable to premature removal of the restoration, which invariably results in the unnecessary loss of additional tooth substance and increases the risk of irreversible pulpal complications. The refurbishment of an old corroded amalgam restoring the occlusal surface of a lower left second premolar tooth is illustrated in Figs 7-3 to 7-5.

Composite Resins

Anterior composite resin restorations require optimum aesthetics. Effective methods of achieving a smooth, well-contoured surface and a high surface lustre are important. Many different abrasive systems are available to help achieve this aim. The most popular methods include polishing discs and strips impregnated with aluminium oxide particles, tungsten carbide finishing burs, finishing diamonds, rubber cups and points impregnated with abrasives and polishing pastes that can be used in association with discs, cups

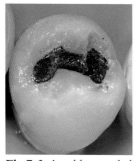 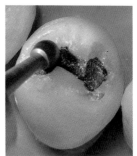 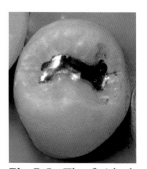

Fig 7-3 An old, corroded amalgam restoring the occlusal surface of a lower left second premolar tooth. The surface is rough and the margins are ditched.

Fig 7-4 Reshaping the old amalgam with steel finishing burs. This procedure should be carried out with water coolant to avoid overheating of the amalgam, minimising the release of mercury vapour, and followed by polishing with abrasive points.

Fig 7-5 The finished, polished amalgam.

and points. Achieving a smooth transition from restoration to tooth without deficiencies or overhangs is of particular importance with composite resin restorations. This avoids unsightly staining of margins in clinical service. If the surface of the composite restoration is rough, it too will attract increased amounts of surface stains. The ability to achieve a smooth surface when polishing a composite resin depends on the:

- finishing system used
- shape of the surface being polished
- size and percentage volume of filler particles within the composite resin
- durability of bond between the filler particles and the matrix
- degree of air inclusion within the bulk of the composite resin, giving rise to porosity.

The smoothest surface on a composite resin is achieved when it cures against a matrix strip, with no finishing or polishing procedures. A range of matrices, strips and crown formers, which can be used to support and shape composite resin as it polymerises, is shown in Fig 7-6. When finishing and polishing is indicated, it is usually achieved using a series of progressively finer discs and, where indicated, strips, with the coarsest discs and strips being used to shape the restorations and the finest to polish the surface.

Abrasive Discs and Strips

Abrasive discs are composed of abrasive particles embedded on a paper or plastic backing. A variety of abrasives may be used, the most popular being aluminium oxide, but silicon carbide and diamond coated discs are also available.

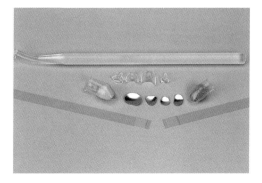

Fig 7-6 Examples of matrices, interproximal acetate strips and crown formers, which can be used to shape and support resin composite, compomer and glass-ionomer cement restorations.

Aluminium oxide discs of various grades of abrasivity give the smoothest surfaces and work best on relatively flat surfaces, such as the labial aspect of anterior teeth. The discs are available in different diameters, ranging from 8 mm to 19 mm, with the smallest discs being useful for accessible sections of gingival margins and proximal surfaces. The discs are used in order of abrasivity: from coarse, through medium, fine and superfine. A range of aluminium oxide discs is illustrated in Fig 7-2. There are differences in the thickness of the discs, with the thinnest being the most flexible and capable of finishing and polishing concave surfaces, such as the palatal/lingual aspects of anterior teeth.

Aluminium oxide discs are mostly used without water coolant in a low-speed handpiece to reduce splatter and increase visibility of the surface to be polished. Running the discs dry results in significant frictional heat. This heat may damage the surface of the composite resin and adversely affect the pulp. Where the tooth surface is convex, for example in cervical restorations, discs have a tendency to flatten the surface. In addition, discs may damage adjacent soft tissues and tooth surfaces, in particular exposed root surfaces, if not used with care. Such damage may be up to 108 µm deep in enamel and 223 µm in dentine. This may compromise the clinical outcome in terms of the appearance of the restored tooth, or give rise to hypersensitivity, which may be difficult to treat (Mitchell et al., 2002).

The discs are held on mandrels. Mandrel design can give rise to aesthetic problems as the head of some mandrels protrudes above the surface of the disc and can be abraded as it is dragged across the surface being polished, leaving unsightly black score marks on the surface of the restoration.

A variation of the aluminium oxide disc is the abrasive-coated finishing strip (Fig 7-2). These strips are useful for removing excess composite from proximal surfaces and, in particular, margins. They are used with a sawing action, being pulled alternately labially then lingually. The strips may be metal or plastic backed. Metal strips are not for the faint-hearted, as they are aggressive to both tooth and restorative material. Great caution must be taken to protect soft tissues when using metal-backed strips. In addition, metal strips are thicker and less flexible than the plastic-backed strips, and, as a consequence, they have a tendency to overcut, leaving surfaces flat and contacts open. They are sometimes used to separate contacts that have inadvertently become bonded together and for orthodontic stripping of proximal surfaces. The majority of metal-backed strips have diamond particles as the abrasive, or less commonly, aluminium oxide. Some metal-backed strips are divided, with a coarse abrasive to one end and a finer abrasive at the other.

Plastic-backed strips are widely used in preference to metal-backed strips, as they are more flexible and less aggressive. Given their flexibility, plastic-backed strips can follow the contour of proximal surfaces apical to the contact area, unlike the more rigid metal-backed strips. Problems may arise, however, if the contact is very tight, as the strip may snag and tear. This can usually be overcome by wedging the teeth apart with a wooden wedge prior to using the strip. Once the strip has cleared the contact, the wedge can be removed to give access to the gingival margin.

Tungsten Carbide Finishing Burs

Tungsten carbide finishing burs are available in a wide range of shapes (Fig 7-7). The number of cutting blades, or flutes, on the finishing burs varies from eight, to 10, 12, 16, 20 and 30, with 12- and 30-fluted burs being the most popular. The bur with the lowest blade count is the most abrasive and is used first, finishing with the bur with the highest blade count. These burs have been shown to produce smooth surfaces when used in conjunction with polishing points. Great care must be taken when using these burs to avoid gouging and otherwise damaging the surfaces of adjacent teeth. Rounded finishing burs are more likely to cause iatrogenic tooth damage than fine-pointed burs. Tungsten carbide finishing burs should be used with water coolant to avoid heat damage and to wash away grinding debris in order to improve visibility and prevent clogging of the flutes. If the flutes of the bur become clogged, the bur will not cut effectively.

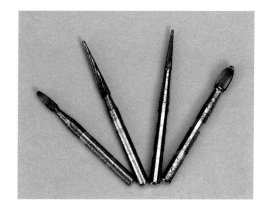

Fig 7-7 Examples of different types of tungsten carbide finishing burs.

Diamond Finishing Burs

Diamond finishing burs are popular for finishing composite resins. They are also used for adjusting and smoothing porcelain restorations and to refine tooth preparations. The burs are available in a wide range of shapes and sizes (Fig 7-8) and with different grits, ranging from 8 μm to 45 μm.

The bur with the largest grit size is the most abrasive and is used first, finishing with the bur with the lowest grit size. Many manufacturers provide coloured rings on the bur shanks to help distinguish the order in which the burs should be used.

The use of finishing diamonds is followed by further refinement and polishing with abrasive-impregnated rubber points or with polishing pastes applied in a prophylaxis cup. Finishing diamonds are best used with water coolant to prevent overheating of the tooth, damage to the surface of the composite and clogging of the abrasive diamond particles by grinding debris.

As with tungsten carbide finishing burs, great care must also be taken when using diamond finishing burs as they can readily damage the tooth surface and soft tissues adjacent to the composite resin restoration. In general, diamond finishing burs give a less smooth surface than tungsten carbide finishing burs and tend to cause more iatrogenic damage.

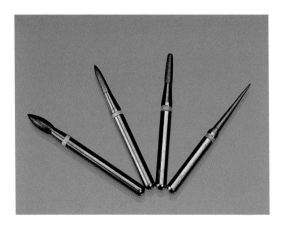

Fig 7-8   Examples of different types of ultrafine finishing diamond burs.

Abrasive-impregnated Cups, Points, Discs and Brushes

A very wide range of abrasive impregnated polymer cups, points, discs and brushes are available for polishing composite resin restorations (Fig 7-9). Cups are a good shape for polishing cusps and slopes in posterior restorations and convex surfaces, notably in cervical restorations. The points are useful for polishing anatomical features such as grooves, fossae and marginal ridges. Brushes can access complex occlusal anatomies. These devices are usually supplied in a kit, with between one and four different grades of abrasive for progressively finishing, polishing and then imparting a high surface gloss. Abrasive particles used include diamond, aluminium oxide and silicon carbide. Some systems are autoclavable, others are disposable for single-patient use. However, many of these items disintegrate rapidly in use, so even if autoclavable, it may be best to consider them as single-use items. In addition, some of these instruments contain latex rubber, with its allergenic potential. These polishing devices are sometimes used in association with polishing pastes to achieve a high surface gloss (Fig 7-9). The pastes contain usually aluminium oxide or fine diamond particles. They are effective, but messy in use.

Surface Sealers

Finishing glosses are available to seal the surfaces and margins of newly placed composite resin restoration. These glosses are usually unfilled or lightly filled photopolymerisable resins which are applied to the surfaces and margins after re-etching the tooth tissues immediately adjacent to the restoration. Some manufacturers produce low-viscosity resins specifically for this purpose, and

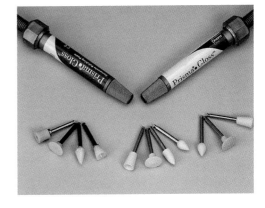

Fig 7-9 A range of abrasive impregnated polymer cups, points and discs are shown in the bottom part of the photograph, with polishing pastes illustrated in the upper part.

these may produce a reduced air-inhibited surface layer compared to alternative low-viscosity resins designed for other purposes, such as fissure sealing.

Surface sealing imparts an aesthetic high gloss to a restoration. It helps seal and mask small defects within the surface of the composite, including air porosities exposed during finishing or microcracks created following the use of finishing devices.

Various other benefits are claimed for surface sealing, including improved marginal integrity, reduced wear rates, decreased surface roughness and less surface staining in clinical service. It is unclear as to whether these benefits are transitory or long-term.

Type of Composite Resin

The smaller the size of the filler particles within the composite resin, the smoother the surface finish will be following finishing and polishing procedures. Smoother surfaces are therefore obtained when microfill, microhybrid and nanocomposite resins are polished, compared with packable or hybrid composites, which include larger filler particles. When composites with larger filler particles are polished, there is a risk that the particles embedded in the surface of the restoration will be dislodged by failure of the silane coupling agent, which bonds the particle to the supporting matrix. When a particle is plucked from the surface, it leaves a defect, adding to the surface roughness of the restoration. The influence of particle size on surface finish and polish is illustrated in Figs 7-10 to 7-13.

Compomers

Compomers have the smoothest surface when set against a matrix. In clinical practice some finishing is invariably required to remove marginal excesses. This must then be followed by polishing, as finishing diamonds and carbide burs leave a relatively rough surface in compomers. In general, polished compomers are much rougher than polished composites.

Manufacturers' directions indicate that compomer restorations can be finished and polished immediately following placement. The evidence supporting this assertion is, however, equivocal, with some workers suggesting that a delay of 24 hours or longer results in a smoother surface and less marginal leakage than subsequent to immediate finishing.

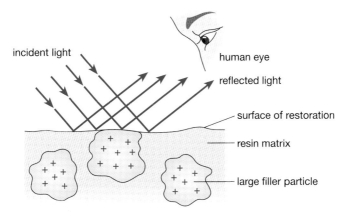

Fig 7-10 The human eye assessing the surface finish and light reflectance of a composite with large filler particles. When newly placed, the surface should appear smooth and shiny.

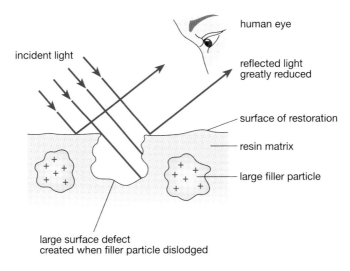

Fig 7-11 The human eye assessing the surface finish and light reflectance of a composite with large filler particles, after a period of wear. One of the large filler particles has become dislodged from the matrix, leaving a large discontinuity in the surface which traps light, reducing reflectance and giving the surface a rough appearance.

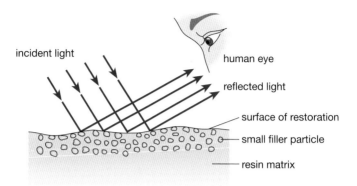

Fig 7-12 The human eye assessing the surface finish and light reflectance of a composite with small filler particles. When newly placed, the surface should appear smooth and shiny.

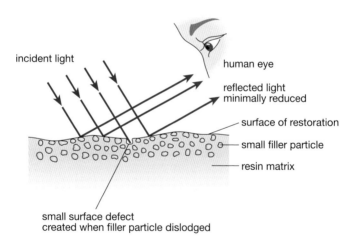

Fig 7-13 The human eye assessing the surface finish and light reflectance of a composite with small filler particles, after a period of wear. One of the small filler particles has become dislodged from the matrix, leaving a small discontinuity in the surface which minimally traps light, with subsequent minimal reduction in reflectance. The surface retains a smooth and shiny appearance.

Glass–ionomer Cements

Conventional glass–ionomer cements are notoriously difficult to finish. On initial setting, the material consists of a delicate matrix of calcium and aluminium polyacrylate salts, containing fluoroaluminosilicate glass filler particles (see Chapter 4, page 56). Glass-ionomers are water-based cements and, as such, are very vulnerable soon after initial set to both dehydration and elution of metal cations required for ionic cross-linking of the material. A delicate balance must therefore be maintained, whereby the relative humidity remains above 80% to prevent dehydration of the cement, while at the same time avoiding exposure to aqueous solutions, such as saliva or water, which will wash away the cations. Clinically, this can be achieved by protecting a newly placed restoration with a matrix as it sets, and coating the surface of the restoration with low-viscosity photopolymerised resin immediately following removal of the matrix. A well-fitting matrix will give the best possible finish to the glass-ionomer cement and limit the amount of subsequent finishing and polishing.

Finishing and polishing is seriously detrimental to the surface and marginal integrity of a newly placed, slow-setting, conventional glass-ionomer cement restoration. Attempts to trim a newly placed glass-ionomer restoration with the use of water coolant results in a weak, chalky surface to the restoration due to elution of cations and insufficient ionic cross-linking. Finishing and polishing should be delayed for at least 24 hours after placement. After this time, finishing and polishing should be carried out with the aid of water coolant to avoid overheating, which damages the structure of the cement.

Instructions for finishing conventional, fast-setting reinforced glass-ionomer cements and resin-modified glass-ionomer cements vary by manufacturer. Some indicate that the material can be trimmed seven minutes after the initial set. The finishing instrument should be lubricated with petroleum jelly or water coolant, dependent on the manufacturer's directions. This approach, however, risks damaging the cement structure. This risk is greatly reduced by delayed finishing.

When finishing restorations of reinforced and resin-modified glass-ionomer cements, the use of rotary abrasives, including aluminium oxide discs, tungsten carbide burs and finishing diamonds, generates excessive heat if used without water coolant. The heat causes water to evaporate from the cement causing shrinkage, which leads to cracking. In addition, the mechanical trauma caused by a rotating instrument physically disrupts the delicate matrix and filler structure of the newly set material. Filler particles are plucked from the surface of the restoration, leaving a relatively rough surface.

References

Mitchell CA, Pintado MR, Douglas WH. Iatrogenic tooth abrasion comparisons among composite materials and finishing techniques. J Prosthet Dent 2002;88(3):320–328.

Oleinisky JC, Baratieri LN, Ritter AV, Felipe LA, de Freitas SF. Influence of finishing and polishing procedures on the decision to replace old amalgam restorations: an in vitro study. Quintessence Int 1996;27(12):833–840.

Chapter 8
Dental Curing Lights

Aim

The aim of this chapter is to improve knowledge of the types of dental curing lights available and their clinical use.

Outcome

Readers will know the relevance of dental curing light irradiance, the advantages and disadvantages of the different types of machine and curing modes available and how to maintain machine performance.

Introduction

Dental curing lights are devices that generate bright light, the energy of which initiates the photopolymerisation of a wide range of light-cured restorative materials. The majority of light-cured restorative materials contain camphorquinone as the photoinitiator. Light with a wavelength of 468 nm is required to initiate polymerisation. A limited number of light-cured materials contain alternative photoinitiators, for example phenyl propanedione (PPD), which requires light with a wavelength of 410 nm to initiate polymerisation (Park et al., 1999). This photoinitiator is sometimes chosen as an alternative to camphorquinone because of its colour stability, which limits "yellowing" of the restoration in clinical service. Alternative photoinitiators are sometimes found in low-viscosity surface sealant materials.

The light output of a curing unit is described as *irradiance*, and is the power output per surface area of the curing tip (mW/cm^2). Irradiance varies between 600 and 2400 mW/cm^2, dependent on the type of curing light used. The amount of energy available to polymerise a material is called the *energy density* – the product of irradiance and time. Therefore, if the irradiance is reduced, it must be compensated for by a longer light exposure time, and vice versa.

Irradiance is reduced under the following conditions:
- low-powered curing light
- larger-diameter curing light guide

- batteries in cordless models in need of recharge
- deterioration in light output of bulb, or ageing, damage or fogging of filters and mirror reflectors
- contamination of curing guide tip by debris, such as polymerised dental materials.

Irradiance can be quantified by means of a radiometer, which is specific for the generic type of curing light. Radiometers can be simple hand-held devices containing a photosensitive diode, or can be built into the curing light. It is recommended that a baseline reading is taken when purchasing a new unit. Irradiance is subsequently checked weekly, and a log kept to determine when it is falling. When a fall in irradiance is detected, steps should be taken to remedy the problem. An alternative method of checking irradiance is to test cure a specimen of dental material in a specially produced mould. In general, these moulds enable an assessment to be made of the depth of material that is being polymerised by the light output. This is a subjective test, which is not always accurate or reproducible; however, it is better than not testing. The output of curing lights can be assessed visually.

The use of a curing light with inadequate irradiance runs the risk of producing restorations with a so-called "soggy bottom" – cured on the surface but still soft at the base. This will lead to early clinical failure, in particular if the "soggy bottom" is located along a cervical margin. Inadequate curing of material will also lead to leaching of uncured resin. This may result in an adverse soft tissue or possibly even a systemic reaction. Other consequences of incomplete curing include increased susceptibility to wear, poor colour stability and possible early breakdown of adhesive bonds.

The energy density required to polymerise a material will increase when:
- The distance from the tip of the light guide to the surface of the material is increased.
- Dark shades of material are used.
- There is polymerisation of certain microfilled composites, which increase light scattering.
- There is polymerisation of flowable composites, which require a higher energy density than hybrid composites.

Under these circumstances, the depth of polymerisation will be reduced and should be compensated for by the placement of thinner increments of material and extending curing times.

Types of Dental Curing Light Available

There is a very wide range of different curing lights available; they vary greatly in cost, number of features, weight, power output and maintenance requirements, among other features. The most commonly used curing lights are:
- halogen light-curing units – also known as quartz-tungsten-halogen or QTH units
- LED (light-emitting diode) units.

Much less commonly used forms of curing units include:
- plasma arc units
- argon lasers.

Halogen Curing Lights

For many years halogen light-curing units were the most common form of curing light in clinical practice. However, LED curing lights are now increasingly replacing halogen units. An example of a halogen curing light is shown in Fig 8-1.

Halogen lights have certain advantages; they:
- are relatively cheap
- have a long, reliable track record
- emit a broad range of light wavelengths (400–510 nm) and are therefore capable of photopolymerising a wide range of light-cured dental materials
- are available in corded or cordless versions.

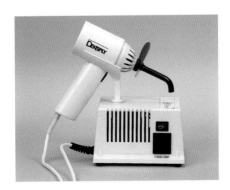

Fig 8-1 Example of a halogen curing light.

The disadvantages of halogen light-curing units include the following:
- The units are inefficient as over 99% of the light output is not in the wavelengths required; this includes light in the infrared range, which generates heat. This heat is in addition to the chemical exotherm created by the cross-linkage of the polymer. Together, these two processes can create unacceptable temperature rises of up to 43.1°C (Al-Qudah et al., 2005). This requires a fan to be included in the unit, which can be noisy and produces hot air, which can be irritating to both the operator and the patient. Fans can continue running for several minutes after light-curing has ceased.
- Some models are relatively bulky, heavy to hold and take up valuable space in the operating area.
- They are lower-output devices than other types of light-curing unit. Overall, this requires exposure time to be longer than with alternative units to ensure appropriate polymerisation.
- The bulb requires periodic replacement.
- Cordless versions require the battery to be recharged relatively frequently.

Halogen curing lights may include the following features:
- Multiple curing modes, such as boost, normal, low, step, ramp and pulse outputs.
- A timer that emits a beep every 10 or 20 s, or a digital display of the time remaining.
- A built-in radiometer, which quantifies light output to check for deterioration of bulb performance.
- A range of sizes of light-curing guides, which can range from 2 to 13 mm diameter. Tips may be disposable, or will require careful decontamination and sterilisation between patients.
- A shield to protect dentists', patients' and dental nurses' eyes from retinal damage by high-intensity light.
- Bulb life ranging from 15 to 100 hours.

Curing Modes
A range of curing modes is available in the more expensive models, while more basic models may only offer one mode.

Boost Mode
On the basis that "time is money", there has always been a drive for dentists to seek faster curing times to increase working efficiency. Thus, more recent halogen curing light units offer a very high output mode for short (<10 s)

exposure times. Application for extended exposure times is likely to result in overheating of the tooth, causing pulpal irritation and pain.

Normal Mode
This is the standard continuous bulb output that may, within reason, be applied for as long as required. Typical exposure times range from 20 to 40 s.

Low Mode
This is a lower output, recommended for polymerisation of thin layers of materials such as dentine bonding agents. Low-mode curing may help to limit stresses created in light-cured materials during polymerisation and generates less heat.

Step Mode
This mode emits a low power output for about 10 s, which then suddenly increases to maximum output for the rest of the curing cycle. The rationale behind this mode is to initiate polymerisation slowly. This is to permit additional time for the material, which becomes rigid as it cures, to deform plastically, relieving stress generated by the shrinkage that accompanies polymerisation.

Ramp Mode
This is a variation of the step mode. In ramp curing the unit emits a low power output for about 10 s, which then increases in a gradual linear manner to maximum output for the rest of the curing cycle.

Pulse Mode
The nature of this mode varies between different units. The power output may be switched on and off for various intervals through the curing cycle, or the output alternates continuously between high and low outputs.

The various curing modes are depicted in Fig 8-2 in terms of their irradiance over time.

Light-emitting Diode Curing Lights

Light-emitting diodes (LEDs) use gallium nitride semiconductors, which emit a blue light through electroluminescence. The light emitted by LEDs has a much narrower spectrum of wavelengths (450–490 nm) than a typical halogen lamp. An example of an LED curing light is illustrated in Fig 8-3. Light output from LEDs is much more efficient than from halogen lamps,

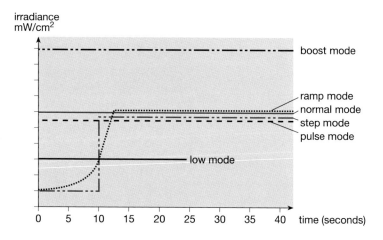

Fig 8-2 Variation of light irradiance over time for various curing modes.

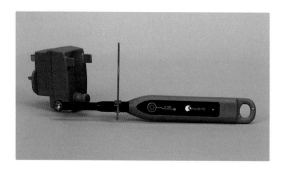

Fig 8-3 Example of a LED curing light and charger unit.

requiring low power consumption and emitting significantly less infrared light – the cause of undesirable heating effects. As a consequence, many LED curing lights do not require a cooling fan, which reduces the bulk and noise output of the unit.

Camphorquinone reacts to light of a wavelength of 468 nm, in the mid-wavelength range of most LED dental light-curing units, but other photoinitiators, found in some photopolymerisable materials such as surface sealants, may not react to this wavelength. Therefore, if using an LED light it is important to check that the materials to be used are compatible with the LED's narrow range of wavelengths. First-generation LED lights were underpowered (Bennett and Watts, 2004), with irradiance levels of 300 mW/cm^2. The irradiance of second-generation LED lights matches that of halogen curing lights. Third-generation LED lights tend to have irradiance levels exceeding those of halogen curing units.

Cordless versions (the majority of models) require recharging of batteries after a time interval ranging between the equivalent of 45 minutes and 2 hours. A fully charged battery can therefore give up to 360 curing cycles of 20 s duration. A fully discharged battery can take up to 2 hours to recharge. It is therefore advisable to purchase two batteries with a unit so that a charged battery is always available.

LED lights have the following advantages:
• They are small and lightweight.
• They are available in corded and cordless versions.
• If cordless, the batteries do not require to be recharged as frequently as those in halogen units.
• There are no bulbs to change.
• There is very low heat generation at the tip of the light guide.
• Fans, if included, are quieter and less of a nuisance than those in halogen units.

However, LED lights have the following disadvantages:
• They may not photopolymerise all materials.
• The selection of light guides may be limited.
• They do not have an established track record.

Plasma Arc Curing Lights

Plasma arc curing units generate light by arcing between two tungsten electrodes in a high-pressure vessel containing xenon gas (plasma). The light output is very powerful and can photopolymerise materials in a much shorter time than light from a halogen or LED curing unit. The wavelength of light output is in the range 380–500 nm. The light is transmitted along fibre optic bundles in the cord that connects the base unit to the light guide. The cord can be stiff and difficult to manipulate and is vulnerable to damage if inappropriately handled. Some models offer extensive preprogrammed curing cycles, for example for photopolymerising through a veneer, or for use during tooth bleaching. Great care must be taken when using plasma arc curing lights as they generate a considerable amount of heat, which can cause pulpal and soft tissue irritation and damage.

Plasma arc curing lights have the following advantage:
• Fast photopolymerisation.

But they have the following disadvantages:
• They are expensive to purchase.
• They are typically larger and heavier than other forms of curing lights.
• There is risk of excessive heat output.

Argon Laser Curing Lights

A laser beam is generated when energy is released through argon gas, creating a high-intensity light. Like plasma arc lights, argon laser curing lights are significantly more expensive than halogen and LED curing lights.

Argon laser curing lights have the following advantage:
• Fast photopolymerisation.

Their disadvantages are:
• They are expensive to purchase.
• They are typically large and heavy units.
• There is risk of excessive heat output.

"Soft-start" Polymerisation

This term is used to describe curing techniques in which the initial phase of light-curing is effected by light of relatively low irradiance. The step, ramp and pulse modes described above for halogen curing lights may be described as "soft-start" methods. These techniques were devised in an attempt to reduce polymerisation contraction and, in turn, reduce polymerisation stresses in light-cured materials in the initial stages of curing. The rationale was that a slower rate of monomer to polymer conversion would enable plastic deformation of the material before it became too rigid, thus reducing shrinkage stress. It was assumed that a reduction in shrinkage stress would correlate with a reduction in susceptibility to leakage, tooth cracking and marginal gap formation and an increase in bond strengths, while maintaining an optimal degree of conversion and hardness.

Soft-start techniques generally do reduce polymerisation stresses; however, this does not necessarily translate into clinical benefits. Indeed, the benefits of soft-start techniques are equivocal. This serves to highlight the fact that the parameter of light-curing varies between curing lights and techniques and according to the material being cured. As in the handling and placement of all materials and in the use of equipment and devices, great care should be taken to understand and strictly apply the relevant directions for use provided by the manufacturers.

Similarly mixed results have been reported for bond strength, degree of conversion and heat generation. It may be that each of these parameters is specific to each type of dental curing light and cannot be generalised across a group, such as halogen or LED light.

Maintenance of Curing Lights

- Check irradiance (light output) weekly with a radiometer.
- Check unit for signs of damage.
- Check end of light guide for debris contamination.
- Keep spare, fully charged battery for cordless models.
- Keep spare bulb for halogen units.
- Ensure that the cooling fan of halogen curing lights has completed its cooling cycle prior to switching off the unit. Prematurely switching off the fan allows halogen gas to be lost from the bulb, allowing oxygen to enter, significantly reducing the life of the bulb.

Risk of Retinal Damage

A curing light must never be directed into a patient's eye. For the operator, it is not advisable to look directly at the high-intensity light emitted by a dental curing light as it can damage the retina. In addition, it can compromise the ability to accurately colour-match tooth-coloured materials to remaining tooth tissues.

Various forms of eye protection are available for both patients and chair-side personnel. These include glasses, goggles, hand-held filters and filters that clip onto the shank of the light guide. Whatever form of eye protection is used, it must be maintained and applied according to the manufacturer's directions.

References

Al-Qudah AA, Mitchell CA, Biagioni PA, Hussey DL. Thermographic investigation of contemporary resin-containing dental materials. J Dent 2005;33(7):593–602.

Bennett AW, Watts DC. Performance of two blue light-emitting-diode dental light curing units with distance and irradiation-time. Dent Mater 2004;20(1):72–79.

Park YJ, Chae KH, Rawls HR. Development of a new photoinitiation system for dental light-cure composite resins. Dent Mater 1999;15(2):120–127.

Chemical Abbreviations

List of Chemical Abbreviations

4-META	4-methacryloxyethyl trimellitic acid
10-MDP	10-methacryloxy decyl dihydrogen phosphate
bis-GMA	bisphenol-A-glycidyl methacrylate
BPDM	biphenyl dimethacrylate
DCDMA	cycloaliphatic dicarboxylic acid dimethacrylate
GDMA	glyceryl dimethacrylate
HEMA	2-hydroxyethyl methacrylate
MAC-10	11-methacryloxy-11-undecadicarboxylic acid
MPAE	methacrylated phosphoric acid ester
MPS	methacryloxypropyl trimethoxysilane
PENTA	dipentaerythritol penta acrylate monophosphate
phenyl-P	2-methacryloxyethyl phenyl hydrogen phosphate
TEGDMA	triethylene glycol dimethacrylate
UDMA	urethane dimethacrylate

List of Dental Manufacturers' Websites

Company name	Global website	UK website
3M ESPE	www.mmm.com	www.3mespe.com/uk
Bisco	www.bisco.com	
Brasseler	www.brasselerUSA.com	
Coltene-Whaledent	www.coltenewhaledent.com	
Cosmedent	www.cosmedent.com	
Danville Engineering & Materials	www.danvillematerials.com	
Den-Mat	www.denmat.com	
Den-Mat Corporation	www.denmat.com	
Dentsply	www.caulk.com	www.dentsply.co.uk
GC	www.gcamerica.com	www.gceurope.com
Heraeus Kulzer	www.heraeus-kulzer-us.com	
Ivoclar Vivadent	www.ivoclarvivadent.us.com	
Kerr	www.KerrDental.com	
Kuraray	www.kuraray.com	
Parkell	www.parkell.com	
Pentron	www.pentron.com	
PulpDent	www.pulpdent.com	
Shofu	www.shofu.com	
Tokuyama	www.tokuyama-us.com	
Ultradent	www.ultradent.com	
Voco	www.voco.com	
Zenith/DMG	www.zenithdental.com	

Index

Quintessentials for General Dental Practitioners Series

in 44 volumes

Editor-in-Chief: Professor Nairn H F Wilson

The Quintessentials for General Dental Practitioners Series covers basic principles and key issues in all aspects of modern dental medicine. Each book can be read as a stand-alone volume or in conjunction with other books in the series.

Publication date, approximately

Clinical Practice, Editor: Nairn Wilson

Culturally Sensitive Oral Healthcare	available
Dental Erosion	available
Special Care Dentistry	available
Evidence-based Dentistry	available
Infection Control for the Dental Team	Summer 2008

Oral Surgery and Oral Medicine, Editor: John G Meechan

Practical Dental Local Anaesthesia	available
Practical Oral Medicine	available
Practical Conscious Sedation	available
Minor Oral Surgery in Dental Practice	available

Imaging, Editor: Keith Horner

Interpreting Dental Radiographs	available
Panoramic Radiology	available
21st Century Dental Imaging	available

Periodontology, Editor: Iain L C Chapple

Understanding Periodontal Diseases: Assessment and Diagnostic Procedures in Practice	available
Decision-Making for the Periodontal Team	available
Successful Periodontal Therapy – A Non-Surgical Approach	available
Periodontal Management of Children, Adolescents and Young Adults	available
Periodontal Medicine: A Window on the Body	available
Contemporary Periodontal Surgery – An Illustrated Guide to the Art Behind the Science	available

Quintessence Publishing Co. Ltd., London